Survival 101 Beginner's Guide 2021

AND

Bushcraft:

The Complete Guide To Urban And Wilderness Survival For Beginners in 2021 (2 Books In 1)

Rory Anderson

Table Of Contents

Survival 101 Bushcraft:
The Essential Guide for Wilderness Survival
2021

INTRODUCTION 3

CHAPTER 1 *WHAT SKILLS DO YOU NEED?* 6

    THE THREE C'S 6

    THE FIVE C'S 8

    THE ORDER OF OPERATIONS FOR SURVIVAL 10

CHAPTER 2: TOOLS YOU NEED 15

    PACKS 15

    CUTTING TOOLS 19

        Swiss Army Knife 19

        Buck Knife 19

        Axe 20

        Saw 20

        Machete 20

        Grind 21

        Whetstone 21

    TYING TOOLS 21

        Rope 21

        Cordage 22

        Snare Wire 22

    LASHING, BINDINGS, AND TOGGLES 22

    COOKING TOOLS 23

        Containers 23

        Pots and Pans 24

        Utensils 24

        Serving Ware 25

BODY COVERAGE TOOLS 26
    Daytime Clothes 26
    Sleepwear 27

CAMP COVERAGE TOOLS 28
    Tarps 28
    Ground Cloths 28
    Rain Covers 29

FIRE TOOLS 29
    Combustion Tools 30
    Fire Starting Materials 30

OTHER CAMP TOOLS 31
    Compass 31
    First Aid Kit 31
    Other Tools 32

CHAPTER 3 *MAKING A SHELTER AND SETTING UP CAMP* 33

THE FIVE W'S OF PICKING YOUR CAMPSITE 33

BUILDING YOUR MAIN SHELTER 35

BUILDING ADDITIONAL SHELTERS 36

TARP SETUP 37
    Flying a Tarp 37
    Tarp Tent 38
    Tarp Lean-To 38
    Diamond Shelter Tarp 39
    Ground Cloth 39

LASHES, BINDINGS, AND TOGGLES 40
    Square Lashing 40
    Simple Binding 41
    Making a Toggle 41

HYGIENE, ORGANIZATION, AND PROTECTION 42

CHAPTER 4 *BUILDING AND MANAGING FIRES* 45

THE TRIANGLE OF FIRE 45

PLACING YOUR FIRE 46

FIRE LAYS 46

The Teepee Fire Lay 46

Log Cabin Fires 47

Long Log Fires 47

Dakota Fire Pits 48

The Cooking Fire Lay 48

STARTING MATERIALS 49

SOURCING WOOD 49

CHAPTER 5 *NAVIGATION AND TRACKING* 51

USING YOUR COMPASS PROPERLY 51

FOLLOWING A MAP 54

THE FIVE NAVIGATION METHODS YOU NEED 56

DETERMINING DISTANCE WHEN TRAVELING 58

FINDING YOURSELF WHEN YOU'RE LOST 59

CHAPTER 6 *SECURING AND STORING FOOD AND WATER* 60

PURIFYING AND STORING WATER 60

PREPARING TO TRAP ANIMALS 61

Signs for Finding Game 62

Bait for Trapping 63

The Components of a Trap 64

Grave's Bait Triggered Snare 65

Fixed Snare 65

Drowning Snare 66

Squirrel Pole Snare 66

Paiute Deadfall 67

Making a Small Trapping Kit for Your Pack 68

    Fishing With Improvised Rods..69

CHAPTER 7 *PROCESSING GAME MEAT* **70**

    Small Mammals...70

    Medium Mammals 71

    Birds 74

    Fish 75

    Reptiles and Amphibians...76

    Cooking Your Meat 77

    Preserving Meat 78

        Drying *78*

        Smoking *79*

    Storing Your Preserved Meat 80

CHAPTER 8 *HYGIENE AND MEDICINE*...**82**

    Personal Hygiene In the Bush..82

    Which Trees and Plants Are Useful...84

    Treating Wounds In the Bush 85

    Dealing With Broken Digits or Limbs 86

    Healing Gastrointestinal Illness In the Bush..87

CHAPTER 9 *LEVERAGING THE ENVIRONMENT*..**88**

    Educating Yourself On Local Plant Life 88

    Properly and Safely Identifying Plants...89

    Consuming and Storing Edible Plants 90

    Using the Landscape to Build a Camp 91

    Getting Creative With the Landscape 92

CONCLUSION **94**

DESCRIPTION **96**

Survival 101 Beginner's Guide 2021:

The Complete Guide To Urban And Wildnerness Survival

INTRODUCTION 99

CHAPTER 1 *PREPARING TO SURVIVE* 102

    GAUGING YOUR CURRENT SITUATION 102

    MEASURING EMERGENCY LEVELS 104

    EMERGENCIES YOU ARE MOST LIKELY TO COME ACROSS 106

    PREPARING FOR EXTREME EMERGENCIES 108

    THE SKILLS YOU WILL NEED 109

CHAPTER 2 *KEY TERMS* 111

    AREA OF OPERATION (AO) 111

    A-TEAM 112

    BUG OUT HIDEOUT SITE (BOHS) 113

    EMERGENCY RALLYING POINT (ERP) 113

    GRAB AND GO BAG (GNG BAG) 114

    IMMEDIATE RALLYING POINT (IRP) 115

CHAPTER 3 *THE FIRST FIVE* 117

    THE FIRST FIVE URBAN VS. OFF-GRID ENVIRONMENTS 117

    SHELTER 119

    WATER 123

    FIRE 124

    FOOD 127

    SAFETY 133

CHAPTER 4 *THE TASK LISTS* 136

    TASKS 1 TO 3: PREPARING 136

    TASKS 4 TO 5: ASSESSING 137

    TASKS 6 TO 12: PREVENTION 138

    TASKS 13 TO 14: COMMUNICATION 140

    TASKS 15 TO 25: THE FIRST FIVE 141

    TASKS 26 TO 27: SPECIAL EQUIPMENT 142

    TASK 28 TO 31: EQUIPMENT CHECKLISTS 142

    TASKS 32 TO 34: LEAVING 143

CHAPTER 5 *THE 34 TASKS OF SURVIVAL* 145

    TASK 1: A-TEAM CONTACTS 146

    TASK 2: WATER BOTTLES 146

    TASK 3: FIRST AID KIT 147

    TASK 4: CHECK STATUS OF A-TEAM 148

    TASK 5: AREA STUDY 150

    TASK 6: FIREARM PREVENTION 151

    TASK 7: FIRE PREVENTION 152

    TASK 8: DROWNING PREVENTION 153

    TASK 9: POISON PREVENTION 154

    TASK 10: ENVIRONMENTAL DANGER ASSESSMENT AND PREVENTION 156

    TASK 11: MAN-MADE DANGER ASSESSMENT AND PREVENTION 156

    TASK 12: MAP AND NAVIGATION SUPPLIES 158

    TASK 13: EMERGENCY RADIO 158

    TASK 14: A-TEAM CODEWORDS 159

    TASK 15: ROTATION AND INSPECTION CHECKLIST 160

    TASK 16: WATER FOR MILD EMERGENCY 161

    TASK 17: WATER FOR MODERATE TO EXTREME EMERGENCY 162

    TASK 18: SHELTER FOR MILD EMERGENCY 163

    TASK 19: SHELTER FOR MODERATE TO EXTREME EMERGENCY 164

    TASK 20: FIRE FOR MILD EMERGENCY 165

    TASK 21: FIRE FOR MODERATE TO EXTREME EMERGENCY 166

    TASK 22: FOOD FOR MILD EMERGENCY 168

    TASK 23: FOOD FOR MODERATE TO EXTREME EMERGENCY 169

    TASK 24: FIRST AID FOR MILD EMERGENCY 170

TASK 25: FIRST AID FOR MODERATE TO EXTREME EMERGENCY 170

TASK 26: EMERGENCY EQUIPMENT FOR WORK/SCHOOL 171

TASK 27: DIGITAL COPIES OF IMPORTANT DOCUMENTS 171

TASK 28: TRAVEL EQUIPMENT 172

TASK 29: SURVIVAL VEST EQUIPMENT 173

TASK 30: PERSONAL EQUIPMENT 174

TASK 31: CAR EQUIPMENT 174

TASK 32: PRE-PACKAGED SUPPLIES 175

TASK 33: GNG BAG FOR MILD EMERGENCY 175

TASK 34: GNG BAG FOR MODERATE TO EXTREME EMERGENCY 176

CHAPTER 6 *HOW TO LEAVE AN URBAN ENVIRONMENT* 177

PREPARING YOUR SUPPLIES 177

PLOTTING YOUR DESTINATION 178

EDUCATING YOURSELF ON YOUR DESTINATION 179

LEARNING SKILLS IN ADVANCE 180

SECURING THE FIRST 5 OF SURVIVAL 181

PRACTICE EVACUATIONS 183

CHAPTER 7 *LONG TERM OFF-GRID SURVIVAL* 185

FORAGING AND SCAVENGING IN NATURAL ENVIRONMENTS 185

RAISED BED GARDENING 186

LONG TERM FOOD PRESERVATION 186

PREPARING FOR CLIMATE CHANGES 187

BUILDING LONG TERM SHELTER 188

NAVIGATING DISASTERS 188

CHAPTER 8 *EMERGENCY AND FIRST AID* 190

WHEN TO CONTACT THE POLICE 190

WHEN TO CONTACT FEMA 191

UTILIZING GOVERNMENT INFRASTRUCTURE 191

FIRST AID METHODS YOU SHOULD KNOW 192

Dressing a Wound	193
Treating a Gastrointestinal Illness	193
Dealing With a Broken Bone	194

CONCLUSION ... 195

DESCRIPTION ... 197

Survival 101: Bushcraft

The Essential Guide for Wilderness Survival 2021

Rory Anderson

INTRODUCTION

What you call bushcraft, others call survival. In the animal kingdom, humans are the only species who have completely eliminated their need to experience a connection to their survival, and it shows. Anywhere you look, you can easily find a society of humans who believe their food comes from the store, their homes come from landlords or the bank, and their means for survival comes from their employer. While this may be true for a modern society, when we get down into the nitty-gritty of survival, this mindset could cost you your life.

Bushcrafting is not a fad, nor is it exclusive to doomsdayers and other conspiracy theorists who believe the world is coming to an end. Bushcrafting is a selection of skills relevant to your survival, that can be used virtually anywhere in the world. When you learn how to preserve your livelihood through survival skills and strategies relevant to the human species, you are no longer at the mercy of our modern society and everything that comes with it. This means when things naturally go wrong, such as pandemics, natural disasters, or economic or political turmoil, you can rely on yourself to survive. With skills that help you survive, such as building shelter, feeding yourself in the wild, and preserving your health and safety, you no longer need to worry about anything that comes your way because you know, for wildfires, that you are prepared.

These days, there's no telling what will happen. Every year, new natural disasters rip through countries, destroying peoples' livelihood and wiping hundreds of thousands of people off the planet. Hurricanes, wildfires, pandemics, disease, and in some cases, even the government are all things you have to beware of when it comes to your survival. More than ever, we are seeing that living in urban environments is dangerous and that you are more likely to be exposed to threats if you live in an urban setting. During situations such as the coronavirus pandemic, for example, people in urban settings are exposed to moderate and extreme conditions, rather than the mild conditions being seen by less busy locales. This increased risk and exposure mean that you may well be required to leave your urban environment should anything go wrong and, if you do, you are going to need to know where to go and what to do once you get there. No matter what it may look like on the surface, we are all just animals looking to survive, and at the end of the day, you can only rely on *one* person to keep you alive – *You*.

Survival 101: Bushcraft is a tell-all book that includes everything you need to know to survive in the wild. From securing shelter and setting up camp to making a fire, navigating, trapping, tracking, and even making your own tools, we are going to cover everything you need to know to live safely and comfortably in the woods for any amount of time. While hobbyists can certainly gain knowledge here, this book was not written to supply some fad-driven industry of people who want to flaunt their knowledge. This book is written to help you survive, no matter what.

I suggest you study this book, keep it on hand, and maintain a hardcopy of it in your survival pack so that if you ever find yourself needing to take to the woods to survive, you have access to everything you need. One thing to know about the human condition is that, under pressure, our memories have a tendency to falter. Rather than placing all that demand on yourself in a circumstance that may already be the most stressful situation you ever face in your life, protect yourself by memorizing the contents of this book and keeping it handy just in case. You never know when you will need this knowledge.

Before you start reading, I want to say thank you for purchasing *Survival 101: Bushcraft*. I know many titles exist on this exact topic already, and I am grateful that you have chosen me to educate you on how to protect your livelihood and the livelihood of everyone you care about.

CHAPTER 1
What Skills Do You Need?

The remainder of this book is going to be focused on clear, step-by-step instructions on how to procure shelter, source, and capture food, and engage in everything else that is required of you in order for you to survive. Before we can get into any of that, though, you need to have a clear understanding of how to actually use any of this knowledge. Without any clear sense of direction or understanding in the order of things, you are going to find yourself struggling to put all of these pieces together to create the ability for you to survive.

Bushcrafting skills require you to control the three C's, core temperature, comfort, and convenience, using the five C's, cutting tools, cover elements, combustion devices, containers, and cordages. The skills you require include things such as making a fire, navigating the wilderness, trapping, foraging, building shelters, making tools, gathering supplies, and improvising as needed. With all of these things put together, you become far more likely to preserve yourself in the wilderness for as long as it is needed.

The Three C's

The 3 C's that are the most important to your survival include core temperature, comfort, and convenience. If either of these three C's are missed when it comes to preserving yourself in the wilderness, you are liable to falter and ultimately fail at surviving in the wild. Protecting these three elements must be your absolute main focus when it comes to establishing your wellbeing and increasing your likelihood of survival.

Core temperature is the primary element that you need to focus on immediately upon entering the wilderness. Especially if it is a cooler season, you need to secure a shelter that is going to be warm enough to maintain a livable body temperature. If your body temperature drops too low, your muscles will begin to stiffen, and it will become much more challenging for you to complete any of the necessary tasks in order to survive. You also run the risk of hypothermia or frostbite. Alternatively, if your body becomes too hot, your blood thickens and you run the risk of heatstroke or dehydration. Under either circumstance, your chances of survival drop drastically, so you need a shelter that helps you maintain a comfortable and manageable body temperature. You will also need clothes or garments you can wear that will provide you with the right body temperature anytime you are leaving the shelter. The clothes you choose, regardless of which climate they are for, need to be flexible enough that you can move around in them so that you can safely complete all of your tasks without your clothes impeding your success.

Your comfort is essential to survival because, to put it simply, without comfort, you begin to lose your will to live. Life may have its challenges and pitfalls, but if you are in a constant state of discomfort, you are going to find yourself coming up against massive amounts of mental, physical, and emotional stress. Physically, stress can damage your ability to maintain enough energy and strength to do everything that is required of you in order for you to survive. Mentally and emotionally, being in a constant state of distress will cause you to lose your will to carry on, which in and of itself can pose a threat to your survival. You must be willing and able to carry on by minimizing your stress as much as possible so that all of your energy can go toward your survival.

Finally, convenience is another essential factor. When you set things up in a way that makes them more convenient for you, you exert less energy into getting things done, which means you are more likely to experience greater levels of comfort. In addition to greater comfort levels, you are also using up fewer calories when things demand less of your energy, which means you do not have to gather as much food to keep up with your energy demands. Further, you can get more done with less amount of time because you are not investing so much into every single task that needs to get done. You will discover that surviving by your own two hands, rather than relying on grocery stores and carefully crafted supply chains, requires a lot more of your time. The more time you can save by making things convenient for yourself, the easier and more enjoyable it will be for you to survive.

The Five C's

The five C's are the tools that are required for you to control your three C's of survival. They include cutting tools, cover elements, combustion devices, containers, and cordages. If all you have are these five things in the wild, you will have plenty to get you started with. Everything else can be made or improvised, while these five things are much more challenging to improvise on and essential to virtually every aspect of surviving in the wilderness.

Cutting tools, including knives, axes, and shears, are all important to have in the wilderness. They will help you build your shelter, harvest and prepare your food, prepare fires, and do many other things that you will find to be essential to your survival. It is a good idea to have a variety of cutting tools on hand, each of which are easy for you to travel with so that you can rely on them as needed. With that being said, you are going to want to opt for multi-tools as they are often space savers, and they tend to be lighter to travel with. For example, a Swiss

Army knife is a great backwoods knife because it can do so many different things, and it is just one single piece of equipment.

Cover elements are useful for many reasons. Cover elements are used to build shelter, cover the ground to give you a cleaner and warmer space to live, and to cover your person so that you remain warm and safe when you leave your shelter. You will also use cover tools to cover and store your food, to pack things around in as needed, and to perform a myriad of other unexpected things when you are in the wilderness. Bringing along as many tarps and other cover elements as you reasonably can is ideal as it prevents you from having to harvest and tan several hides to build a shelter in. While there is room for improvising in the wilderness, you should still have some basic man-made cover elements, too.

Combustion devices are necessary as they allow you to start a fire. You may have seen different programs on TV where people strike flint and other elements together to make fire, and while this does work, it also takes a lot of time. Further, not every environment has minerals in it that are capable of starting fires. Ideally, you want to bring along as many matches as you possibly can, all in water-proof bags to prevent them from getting wet and not working any longer. You should also bring along lighters and lighter fuel, if possible, as they will be helpful in starting fires, too. Another excellent device that was recently developed is known as a permanent match, and it is a single tool that can be used over and over again to start a fire. This is a great tool to have on hand as it will help you keep your fire going for as long as possible.

Containers are useful in survival when it comes to storing food and water. You want containers that can be properly cleaned so that you are able to safely store everything inside of them without the worry of bacteria getting in and damaging the quality of your food or water. Ideally, you should use stainless steel containers as they can safely be boiled to eliminate bacteria, and are less likely to harbor bacteria in the first place. Plus, they are rust-resistant so they will last significantly longer. For water, purchasing a self-filtering water bottle is a good idea, too. Many survival stores sell self-filtering stainless steel water bottles that are capable of eliminating any contaminants from water found in the wilderness. This is a sure way to protect yourself against harmful bacteria that could lead to disease and, possibly, death. While plastic may seem easier and more accessible in our modern society, note that plastic harbors bacteria, and it cannot be boiled to clean it properly, which makes this a poor choice for bushcraft.

Cordages, or types of rope and cord, are important for your camp, too. You are going to want to bring along as much rope as you can in four different weights. You need a thread and needle for sewing, a lightweight nylon or paracord rope for hanging tarps and doing other similar tasks, a medium weight rope for building snares and traps, and a heavyweight rope for a variety of uses, from hanging food to helping you haul things around if need be. You should bring along as many lengths of each rope as is possible, as rope will always come in handy on a campsite.

The Order of Operations for Survival

Survival requires five basic things to be fulfilled: oxygen, water, food, shelter, and self-defense. When you can fulfill these five needs, you have everything you require in order to survive. Everything thereinafter is to create an easier means of survival for yourself. With that being said, if these five things are not fulfilled in the proper order, you will create vulnerabilities within yourself, which can threaten your survival. It is crucial that you follow the right steps to secure all five of these things as fast as possible, and as efficiently as possible so that you can guarantee your survival.

Although there are only five things that are required in order for you to survive, there are actually ten steps that need to be taken in order for you to survive. You must take these ten steps in order to ensure that you are ready to face the challenges that lie ahead of you. Understand that all ten of these things must be fulfilled in every single emergency, no matter how large or how small that emergency may seem. In some scenarios, you may be able to secure certain aspects of your survival through urban means, while in others, you may need to be solely responsible for procuring the supplies and building your own means of survival. You should be prepared to do whatever it takes, in any situation, to ensure your safety and the safety of anyone with you.

The first order of operations when it comes to survival is to get yourself in the mindset of surviving. When you first find yourself in a situation where you are solely responsible for your survival, it can come as a shock, and it can leave you feeling terrified, and even feeling like a victim of your circumstances. If you stay in this mentality, however, you are going to struggle to take charge and take the necessary action because you will be overridden by fear. As soon as you find yourself in a situation where you need to be responsible for your survival, you need to focus on staying as positive as you possibly can so that you can secure your means of survival. Positivity is going to boost your resiliency, your creativity, and your overall mental toughness so that it is easier for you to endure anything that comes your way.

The second order of operations is to render first aid. As you are leaving an urban environment, bring along as many first aid items as you possibly can. Ideally, you should have a fully equipped medical kit ready to go in case you ever find yourself in a survival setting, that way you can grab it and take it with you as a part of your supplies. We will discuss the exact tools you need in greater depth in Chapter 2: Tools You Need.

The third order of operations is to consider how you are going to defend yourself should anything go wrong. Knives and axes are incredibly helpful when it comes to self-defense. If you are capable of owning a gun and enough ammo and bringing it with you, this can be another great tool for self-defense. Be sure to use safety and transport of any sort of weaponry safely to avoid accidental injury or death.

The fourth order of operations is to make sure you have signals for every single person in your camp. While this will not necessarily be used third, before you leave an urban environment, you will want to secure whistles for each person who will be in your camp. As long as you can breathe, whistles will help you call for assistance to anyone else who may be in the bush with you, so they are important. This way, should you find yourself in danger or injured in the bush, you can signal to each other and receive prompt help.

Once you get into the bush itself, you reach the fifth order of operations. That is, to build a shelter. You need to build a shelter as fast as you possibly can, as nightfall will come, and temperatures will drop. While you can generally go about three days without water and about three weeks without food, it takes just a few hours for hypothermia and frostbite to settle in. Building a shelter will ensure that you have a safe, warm place to stay so that you do not find yourself exposed to the elements and damaging your potential to survive.

The sixth order of operation is to get water. You do not want to start a fire and then leave camp, and water will be needed rather quickly. If you were unable to bring any with you, you are going to want to find a safe water source like a stream, a river, or a waterfall to get water from. You are going to need to sterilize the water before drinking it, so unless you have a bottle that conditions water on the spot, wait until you are back at camp to safely do so.

The seventh order of operation is to build a fire. Once you are safely back at camp with your water, you can build yourself a fire so that you have warmth. Fire will also help you maintain light in the evening, boil water, cook food, and dry out your clothes if need be. You should have fire-starting materials on your person at all times so that if you ever get stuck away from the camp you have made; you can make yourself a fire. You should also have a fire going as often as possible at camp, ideally with someone there to tend to it to keep it from going out. It is easier to find wood to maintain a burning fire than it is to find more combustion tools to start a new one, so you want to preserve your fires for as long as possible to minimize your usage of combustion tools.

When shelter, water, and fire have been secured, you need to move on to food. Food is your eighth order of operations, and it should be found within 24-48 hours, especially since you will be stressed out, and your body needs food to help it remain resilient against everything you are up against. While you may be able to survive 3 weeks without food, the longer you go without it, the harder it will be to have enough energy to source any food. Food will be an all-consuming task since you are going to need to eat multiple times per day, so you should be ready to set up multiple means for securing food sources. Fishing, trapping, and foraging are all great places to start as they can provide you with easy access to nutritional food sources. When you are preparing your food, make sure you wash and cook it thoroughly to avoid accidentally ingesting any bacteria that may cause you to get sick, as curing sickness in the wilderness can be rather challenging, and it can pose a major threat to your survival.

The ninth order of operations is to keep yourself motivated. Especially if you are not used to having to be so hands-on with your survival, it can be easy to want to give up and throw in the towel. The amount of stress you face from a massive change in circumstances and the requirements of surviving can be exhausting and can prove to be a major burden. The longer you go on, the more you may wish to give up. This can worsen in the earliest hours of the morning, around 2 A.M., when your brain chemistry dips and pain levels become worse, and thoughts become darker and more challenging to face. If you can get yourself through the nights, getting through the days will be easier, and surviving will become more achievable.

The tenth order of business is to rescue yourself. In an ideal scenario, you would be able to use smoke signals to indicate where you are at so that a chopper can locate you, and you can be rescued. And, in some emergencies, that may still be required of you, so you will want to maintain a large enough fire that you can be located. If, however, you know that you are unlikely to be rescued, you are going to have to rescue yourself. This means that you are either going to need to find your way into a civilization where you can stay, or you are going to need to create your own civilization where you can stay indefinitely until things change. It may seem like an impossible thing to do, but where there is a will there is a way, and if you can stay on track with securing your survival, you will find a way.

CHAPTER 2: TOOLS YOU NEED

Living in civilized society at present means that you have access to many tools that would be virtually impossible for you to source in the bush. Sourcing and storing tools that will aid in your survival is important, as it allows you to have everything handy should you find yourself in an emergency survival situation. In this chapter, we are going to discuss all of the different tools you should source and keep handy so that you can take these with you if need be. It is important that you get the best possible tools for yourself that are going to be the most useful in a survival situation. It is also important that you do not have too many things as you have to think in terms of practicality, including how practical it will be for you to transport everything. You want to bring only the most necessary things so that you can survive, as you will be able to source everything else from the bush.

When it comes to bushcrafting, you'll note that there is no "one" tool in any given category that is *the* best. Rather, there are many great tools out there, and you are going to need to find the ones that are most accessible for you. Get the best of what you can afford, and the one that is going to be easiest for you to handle and make use of, while also having the strength and longevity it needs to endure life outdoors for extended periods of time. That way, you know you are investing your money in a worthy investment.

Packs

Packs are a crucial tool when it comes to bushcrafting. You need a pack that is going to give you enough room for all of your supplies, while also distributing the weight evenly across your back so that it is easy for you to carry those supplies. Packs made for bushcrafting have an ergonomic aspect to them to make them easier to carry for longer periods of time, and they are made to be hardy and lightweight so that they can endure the bush without adding excess pounds to your luggage.

There are ten different elements you are going to need to consider when it comes to buying the right pack, and these elements are best looked for in person so that you can feel confident in the pack you are buying. With that in mind, do your best to avoid purchasing your pack online as it could lead to an expensive and poor quality purchase.

First, you need to consider the size of the back that you need. Hobbyists and weekend campers can get away with smaller packs, but if you plan on surviving in the woods for any period of time, you are going to need as large of a pack as you can manage. If you have other members of your household that will be coming with you, you want to fit each of them with a pack they can carry, too, so that you can transport more with you.

Next, you need to consider where the frames are within the pack. External frames are old-school packs that were used by previous generations, though they are not as popular as they once were because they can cause pressure sores on the various areas where they touch the body. However, they do allow you to carry more inside of the pack and strap gear outside of the pack because of where they are situated. Internal frames, on the other hand, may be more comfortable to carry, but they do take up more space in the pack and eliminate your ability to strap as many things to the outside of your pack. Another thing to consider is where you are likely to end up. External frames can be bulkier, so if you think you will end up in overgrown brush, an internal frame would be better as it will be easier for you to carry through the bush.

Hip belt and shoulder padding are important features to consider. The majority of the weight of your pack will sit on your hips, and much of it will be in your shoulders, too. Packs with added padding in these two areas can be more comfortable to carry, especially if you suspect you will need to carry them for a long way, as they will relieve some of the pressure off of your hips and shoulders.

Proper ventilation on a bushcraft pack is important, no matter what weather you think you are likely to be in when you are carrying your pack. Your pack will create heat against your back, and in warmer conditions, this will be especially uncomfortable. This heat can also lead to sweating and sores, which can both be dangerous, depending on the situation. A properly ventilated pack should be made of mesh, which will help you regulate body temperature more efficiently.

External attachments are essential when it comes to a pack that will be used in survival circumstances. External attachments ensure you can strap more to your pack as needed so that you can carry more with you. Look for a pack with a variety of external attachments so that if you need them, you have them.

Bushcraft packs need to be well-organized when you pack them so that you can find everything easily, so you need a pack that has different access points and organized compartments. With that being said, packs with more compartments can be more expensive, so don't go overboard. Buy what you can afford, as you can always take care of organization through other methods later on, such as using smaller storage bags inside.

Especially if you live in a wet climate, you are going to want a pack with a rain cover. With core temperature being as important as it is, the last thing you want is to arrive at camp and have everything too wet for use. A rain cover will keep everything inside your pack dry. You can either buy a pack that has one built-in, or you can buy a separate rain cover for your pack. Be sure to keep it in an easily accessible spot in case you need to use it.

Packs with removable lids are handy as these lids can help you store more within the pack, but they can also be removed and left behind to reduce weight as needed. If you will be living in the bush for an extended period of time, this is helpful as you can offload many of your belongings at camp and pack just what you need for shorter trips away from camp, such as when you are hunting or fishing for the day.

Built-in water reservoirs can be extremely helpful in packs, especially if you are able to fill your pack with water before you leave your home. This way, you have safe drinking water as you prepare camp for the days, weeks, or months ahead. If your pack does not have a hydration system in it, do your best to fill water bottles and pack them before leaving so that you have access to clean, fresh drinking water.

Finally, you need to check that the pack fits you. Packs come in all shapes and sizes, and some are going to fit while others will not. Try the pack on, put some weight in it, and walk around a bit to see if it is comfortable. Finding a pack that fits you properly is important, as a well-fit pack is easier to carry for longer periods of time. This way, you are able to preserve your comfort and your energy levels, making bushcraft much easier for you.

Cutting Tools

Cutting tools are essential in a survival situation. You will use them to cut down branches to help build your camp, to chop wood so you can build fires, to cut your tying tools with, to cut your food with, and to do so many other things with. Proper knives, axes, and saws, as well as sharpening tools, will be important for your camp. Ideally, you should have the following four types of cutting tools: a Swiss Army knife, a buck knife, an ax, and a saw. If you can bring a machete or a similar size knife with you, this will also be helpful. You can add more knives if you feel it is needed, such as ones to eat with or additional knives for additional members who will be coming with you. Otherwise, these will be enough to keep you going.

Swiss Army Knife

Swiss Army knives, with all of their ends and attachments, are useful when bushcrafting. Ensure you buy a high-end Swiss Army knife with a proper grip on it made of high-quality wood or stainless steel to ensure that it is likely to last. Low-quality knives like ones made of plastic will fall apart quickly, rendering them useless. Ideally, every adult member of your camp should have a Swiss Army knife as they can be used for so many things.

Buck Knife

Buck knives are great for hunting, particularly when it comes to butchering the animals you harvest. A buck knife is a heavier duty knife that can be used for many purposes as well, including cutting thicker ropes with, cutting smaller branches with, or even whittling branches into arrowheads so they can be used to spear fish if needed. While a buck knife with a fixed handle may be more durable, one that can be flipped closed for storage is safer to carry around in a pack. If you get one with a fixed handle, be sure to get a proper sheath to avoid accidentally cutting yourself on the knife.

Axe

Axes are great when it comes to building camp, and building fires. You will be able to cut back smaller pieces of wood as well as make firewood as needed. In the event of an emergency, axes can also be wielded as a weapon in case of a wild animal invasion on your campsite.

Saw

Saws will be excellent for building camp. With a saw, you can cut back pieces of wood and fashion them into various shapes to help you build shelters, tables, chairs, and other camp necessities. They are excellent building tools, and therefore are incredibly handy to have on a campsite. You should have a single-handled saw that is large enough to cut through large logs, but small enough to transport into the bush. Make sure the blade is cut of stainless steel or a similar metal to ensure they are rust-proof, as you will want your saw to last a long time. As well, opt for a handle made of treated wood or comfortable metal so that it will last in the bush, too.

Machete

If you will be going into an overgrown forested area, a machete is an excellent tool to use to help you whack back branches and carve out paths for yourself. You can also use it to cut back any overgrowth that may be growing into your campsite. As well, machetes can be used as a weapon when needed, so it is a good idea to keep it close by, especially when you are sleeping. This way, if you find yourself under attack, you can protect yourself and your campsite.

Grind

Grinds are a sharpening tool that can be used to sharpen any knife blade as needed. It is a good idea to keep a grind on hand at all times so you can sharpen your blade, as sharp blades are less dangerous than dull or chipped blades. Grinds are generally an easier sharpening tool to use, as they have a cutout in them where the knife is inserted to perform the sharpening process. You should have at least one for your campsite.

Whetstone

Whetstones are another type of sharpening tool that can be used to help sharpen any blades you have with you at your campsite. With whetstone, you will need to first dampen it, and then you will need to drag the blade on a 15-degree angle back toward yourself, with the sharp end of the blade pointed away from you. This will help you sharpen the knife and clean off any chips that may occur on the sharp edge of the knife, thus keeping your knife safe to be used.

Tying Tools

Tying tools will be used for everything from creating snares and safely storing food above the ground, to tying up tarps and tying branches together to create shelter. Tying tools can also be used to tie pelts and hides together so that you can create more cover elements, or even to help carry things through the woods. These incredibly versatile tools come in handy more than you might expect, so you will need a healthy variety for your campsite.

Rope

Because of how much tying you will be doing in the bush, it is important that you have tying materials that are strong, durable, and easy to work with. Layered sisal rope is a great option for rope, as is paracord. While neither will be functional for climbing purposes, they will both be strong enough to perform many other duties that assist in your survival.

For climbing purposes, you want something that is around 9.5mm and made of something that is intended for climbing. Generally, climbing ropes are made of nylon fibers that are wound tightly together, and they feature a nylon sheath, so that they are strong, durable, and can be rubbed against any surface without tearing and dropping you in the process.

Cordage

Cordage varies from rope to rope in that it is made of a set of ropes and cords, while ropes are made of thick strings and fibers that come together to make them stronger. Paracord, Dyneema, and ultra-high molecular weight polyethylene (UHMWPE) are all great cordages that can be used in your camp for a variety of purposes. Nylon cords are also great as, much like with climbing rope, they are made in such a way that causes them to be incredibly durable.

Snare Wire

Snare wire is a specific type of wire that is used to create snares which are used to catch small mammals such as rabbits and hares. This wire is thin and clear so that animals cannot see it, and it is set in areas where the animals are likely to run through so that as they run through, the snare catches them. Once they are caught by the snare, they will pass away, which will make harvesting them and bringing them back to camp easier.

Lashing, Bindings, and Toggles

Lashing, bindings, and toggles are actually skills rather than specific tools; however, they are used as tools when it comes to bushcrafting. All three of these skills are forms of knot skills that use cordage and rope to help you create a certain desired effect with your rope. Lashing is a rope strategy that forms a web of sorts that connects a variety of things together, such as large branches for a fence or for shelter. Lashing is not so much of a true knot form as a wrap that is used to hold things together. Binding is similar to lashing, except it contains fewer wraps because it is only intended to hold something snuggly together, like a true knot. Finally, toggles are a moveable crosspiece that is used to connect or fasten something together. A simple example of a toggle would be if you were to make yourself a poncho and connect it at the front by a rope loop on one side with a small stick on the other side that would be inserted through the rope loop to hold both ends of the poncho together. These toggles can be used in a variety of different methods in bushcraft and can be made in a variety of different sizes, too.

Cooking Tools

Securing food is going to be an ongoing process when you are in the bush, and so is cooking that food since you are going to need to be absolutely confident that your food is safe to eat. Especially when it comes to game meat, you need to ensure that the meat is thoroughly cooked all the way through every single time to avoid ingesting anything that could contain diseases or parasites, which would make you sick and possibly kill you.

Containers

You will see a great deal about what types of containers to use for bushcraft, ranging from different types of plastic containers to plastic bags and even old plastic food containers such as clean plastic peanut butter jars. While these may be effective for hobbyists or short term bushcrafters, they will not be ideal for long term survival as they can quickly become filled with bacteria and challenging to properly cleanse in the bush.

Stainless steel food containers and water canteens or other metal containers with properly securing lids that are completely rust resistant and capable of tolerating high temperatures are best when it comes to storing food. These types of containers can easily be boiled for sterilization so that they can be reused over and over again. Glass can also be used, though it will be heavier and a little more dangerous to transport due to the fact that it could break. As well, if a glass container cracks, you will not be able to use it any longer as the cracks will harbor bacteria.

Pots and Pans

Cast iron and stainless steel cookware are the best options when you are living in the bush. Be mindful that cast iron can be rather heavy, so bringing along only one or two cast iron cookware items is ideal to avoid having to carry anything excessive into the bush. Stainless steel pots are excellent as they can handle virtually anything, can be properly sterilized, and will not rust in the bush.

Avoid anything with a non-stick coating, as non-stick coatings break down over an open flame, and over certain temperatures. They can quickly contaminate your food and cause you to become sick, which is obviously not ideal.

In addition to pots and pans, you may want to get yourself a cast-iron kettle, or a stainless steel kettle that you can take with you. While water can be boiled in a pot for drinking purposes, boiling it in a kettle makes it easier to pour into your drinking containers.

Utensils

Cooking utensils are important when it comes to bushcraft as you do not want to risk putting your hands anywhere near hot water, hot cookware, or hot food. Burns may seem minor in an urban environment, but in the bush, they can quickly become infected which can lead to a life-threatening situation.

Wooden and rust-resistant metal utensils are optimal. Choose barbecue-sized utensils when it comes to tongs, spatulas, and other cookware that will be used directly over the fire as they will afford you more space between your hand and the flame. Select a few different types of spoons, tongs, a spatula, and a stainless steel mesh sieve for your bushcraft utensils. You should also bring along a pair or two of oven mitts, though keep in mind that they need to be used very cautiously around the fire as they can catch fire, and they only work up to certain temperatures.

Another cooking tool you may wish to have on hand is a large metal S hook. When cooking in the bush, your oven mitts may not be useful, and you are going to need a way to remove your pots from the oven. An S hook can be inserted through a handle and used to carefully remove a hot pot or pan from the top of your oven, so long as there is not too much inside of that pot or pan which could lead to splashing and burns.

Serving Ware

As with the rest of your cookware, stainless steel serving ware is the best option as it gives you the ability to properly sterilize your dishes between meals. Only bring one plate, one bowl, and one fork, spoon, and knife per person camping with you. You might bring one additional set just in case, but otherwise, you will be wasting space and weight on serving ware. Be sure to clean them thoroughly between meals to avoid contamination and sickness.

Body Coverage Tools

When it comes to surviving in the bush, it can be easy to think about what tools you will need to help you build shelter, harvest food, and cook the food. However, you may not think about clothing until the last minute. Nonetheless, clothing is imperative as you need clothes that are going to help you maintain the proper body temperature while also being practical and useful. As with everything else, you want to avoid bringing too much, so opt for clothes that are going to be functional and practical when it comes to survival situations.

Daytime Clothes

For daytime clothes, you will want two pairs of pants, two short sleeve shirts and two long sleeve shirts, a proper survival jacket, at least three pairs of underpants, and eight pairs of long socks.

For your pants, opt for khaki cutoff style pants that can easily be transformed into a pair of shorts, as this will help you maintain your temperature in both hot and warm climates without taking up nearly as much space in your pack.

For your jacket, opt for one that has an inner shell that can be removed and used as a sweater on days when an entire jacket may be too heavy. The outer shell of your jacket should have plenty of pockets that you can use to store various survival items, ranging from a small on-the-go first aid kit to snacks and your Swiss Army knife.

For your socks, opt for four pairs of cotton socks for hotter days and four pairs of wool socks for cooler days. Packing plenty of socks is important as these are the first clothing items to wear down in the bush due to all of the walking you will be doing, so you want plenty of extras.

For everything else, opt for breathable yet durable clothes made of cotton. Avoid clothing brands that are known for quickly breaking down and opt instead for brands that can withstand the outdoors so that your clothing is more likely to last you. Making your own clothes in the bush can be rather challenging, so you want to avoid finding yourself in any such situation.

If you are going to be in a particularly cool climate, you may also want to bring a pair or two of thermal underwear, which can be worn under your clothes for added warmth. Thermal underwear made of a wool blend will be best as it will be breathable while also helping to keep you warm.

Sleepwear

Your sleepwear should always be separate from your daytime clothes, as you want something clean, dry, and warm to sleep in. Not only will this support you with survival, but it will also help boost morale by helping you feel more comfortable when you rest. Thermal underwear is a great choice for sleeping, though light cotton pants and shirts can be used, too. You should opt for full pants and long sleeves with your sleepwear, as this will help ensure that you are keeping yourself protected. Exposed skin is exposed to bugs that can carry bacteria and disease, so you want to avoid being exposed whenever possible.

In addition to actual clothes, be sure to bring a sleeping bag for each person that will be staying with you. You will want to get one that is durable, and that can withstand cold temperatures so that if you find yourself out below freezing, you will have everything you need to survive.

Camp Coverage Tools

Coverage for your camp is equally as important as coverage for your body, as it will give you an extra layer of protection from the elements. While much of your coverage can be crafted from brush and branches, having man-made coverage tools can help ensure that your camp is far more protected by offering better shade and water protection.

Tarps

Tarps will always be helpful when you are bushcrafting. Ideally, you should have one small, one medium, and one large tarp. You may also want to bring one additional small tarp to be used for patchwork on your other three tarps, should they begin to tear. Otherwise, the small tarp can be used over small areas, or it can be used to help protect your food reserves. Medium and large tarps can be used in the building of actual shelters to minimize your exposure to the eliminates.

You want to avoid using brightly colored tarps as they can attract attention to your camp and encourage unwanted animals to visit you. Instead, choose neutral colors that will blend in with the environment you will be in so that you can protect yourself from wildlife.

Ground Cloths

Ground cloths are used to help protect you from the elements below you. The ground itself can harbor bugs, bacteria, and a lot of moisture, especially if you are in a more humid or wet climate. Bringing along ground cloths can protect you from those elements by giving you a layer of protection between yourself and the bare ground.

You can choose tarps for ground cloth, though you will also want to have warmer, thicker options to place over your tarps. While tarps will keep away moisture and provide an additional layer to protect you from bugs, waxed canvas and animal hides are also great. Waxes canvas aids in protecting you against moisture in the ground while also providing an additional layer for warmth, while animal hides will add warmth and cushion, particularly for areas where you will be sleeping.

Rain Covers

Tarps are great for rain covers, though waterproof canvas, nylon, felt, and polyester are all great, too. These are all materials that are commonly used to make waterproof tents with, and they can be used for a number of things from keeping yourself dry to keeping areas of your camp protected from the rain. If you have enough space in your pack, and you know you live in a climate that is generally wet, these materials can be used to cover common walkways in your camp to keep you dry from place to place. For example, between your sleeping shelter and your cleaning shelter. This way, you are able to keep yourself dry and comfortable the entire way. Again, choose neutral colors that will not attract any attention from neighboring wildlife.

Fire Tools

Fire is essential to survival, so you are going to want to pack plenty of things to help you aid in building and maintaining fires in your camp. Combustion tools as well as starter materials will be important as they all provide you with what you need to create and maintain a fire. Actual firewood can be harvested from the bush itself, so do not worry about that.

Combustion Tools

In bushcraft, there are three types of combustion tools you can use: matches, lighters, and permanent matches. Matches are often inexpensive and are easy to travel with, so pack as many as you can, as well as match striking material so you can start your matches. Be sure to store them in a double-wrapped, heavy-duty waterproof zip-locked bag to avoid any moisture getting into your matches.

Lighters are also great for bushcraft, though they can die out once the fuel has been used up, so you may want to keep added fuel on hand. Barbecue lighters, as well as cigarette lighters, are best for bushcraft, as barbecue lighters can be used for larger fires in your camp while cigarette lighters can be used for smaller ones when you travel away from camp, such as for hunting.

Permanent matches are devices that were made specifically for bushcrafting, and they are designed to start your fire over and over again without requiring anything aside from the permanent match itself. Keeping one or two on hand is an excellent choice for bushcrafting as they are reliable, efficient, and can be used for a long time, while matches and lighters will eventually run out.

Fire Starting Materials

When you want to get a good fire going, you are going to need a lot more than some well-placed logs to get you started. You need materials that are going to quickly catch fire so that you can keep the fire going long enough to catch your wood on fire. Cotton, dryer lint, pine cones, wood shavings, and dry grass are all excellent fire-starting materials that are lightweight and easy to travel with, and some of them can even be found right there in the bush. You will want to keep plenty on hand so you can start and maintain your fires as needed.

Other Camp Tools

There are a few additional camp tools you should have on hand that will help you survive in the bush for any period of time. These tools may not belong to any particular category, but they are important to your survival.

Compass

A good lensatic compass for bushcrafting is one that is properly set and reliable. You may even wish to have two on hand to ensure that you are able to keep exact track of yourself while you are traveling away from camp. Choose a functional and practical compass made of a rust-resistant metal that will work for years to come, and practice using it, so you know exactly what to do when it comes time to rely on it.

You should also keep several pieces of paper and writing tools on hand, including pencils and colored pencil crayons, as you can use them to help you create a map of your surroundings so that you know exactly where you are at all times. Keeping track will be important, as you never want to venture so far away that you end up lost and without any of your survival tools.

First Aid Kit

Your first aid kit should be filled with gloves, drugs, and medications, antiseptic wipes, minor wound and blister kits that include gauze, steri-strips, a suture kit, wound dressing pads, plasters, compeed, and a thermometer, a crepe bandage, a military dressing or two, a nasopharyngeal airway, a syringe, a blunt needle, a CPR mask, small bandages, transpore tape,

Betadine, benzoin, a temporary cavity or tooth filling, superglue, tweezers, safety pins, a whistle, sheers, a lighter, and a head-torch. If you have a child on hand or access to one or two diapers, you should include these in your medical kit, too, as they are excellent for absorbing blood should a more intense wound be sustained. You should also have a write up of important usage factors, such as any important information on the drugs and medications, and instructions on how to use the plasters and apply the bandages. This way, you know exactly what to do and how to use them without causing damage to the person you are applying these tools on.

Other Tools

In addition to everything previously mentioned, you will want to bring anything else you can that will help you with survival. Binoculars, fishing line, and hooks, a shovel, baskets, additional filters for water filtration, flares, a radio, solar-powered flashlights, a small sewing kit with extra sewing needles, a mallet, and a metal grate for cooking on top of are all great tools to have on hand, also.

CHAPTER 3

Making A Shelter And Setting Up Camp

As you know, the first order of operations upon arriving in your area of intended survival is to set up camp. You are going to need a single shelter, first, which will be used as a primary shelter for sleep, storing your belongings, and changing your clothes, as well as hiding away from the elements as needed. After you have built your initial shelter, you will go on to create any additional shelters you need for your camp, ranging from a separate place to store your goods, a place to safely store your foods, a place to cook, and a place to practice hygiene.

The Five W's of Picking Your Campsite

Where you set up camp is just as important as how you set up camp, as the location of your camp will aid in convenience and comfort, as well as your ability to maintain a proper core temperature. There are five W's that you need to consider when it comes to picking the right campsite, including water, waste, weather, widowmakers, and wildlife.

Your camp should be close to water so that you can easily haul water back to camp without having to trek too far to get it. However, you do not want to be so close to water that you run the risk of being caught in a flood zone. Look for a spot that will be higher than the water itself, yet close enough that it is easy for you to access.

Waste removal will be important for your campsite as it ensures hygiene while also keeping possible wildlife attractants away from you. Ideally, you should pick a waste removal spot that will allow you to easily package and remove waste from the woods when you are ready to leave. However, that may not be practical if you will be surviving there for an extended period of time.

For that reason, simply choose somewhere farther away and easy to access. As well, make sure your waste is not upstream from where you are, and that it is not at risk of contaminating your water in its final location.

Weather is one of your biggest risk factors when it comes to survival, regardless of how nice the weather seems. It can turn fast, and any type of weather can be particularly challenging to navigate when you are exposed. Pick an area that offers natural shelter, and that will not run the risk of exposure to things such as wind and precipitation.

Widowmakers are a type of tree. Specifically, they are a dead tree that is already beginning to dry off and rot. A strong gust of wind or any heavy precipitation can lead to these trees falling over, which can be incredibly dangerous for your camp. In some instances, they have even been responsible for major injury and death. You want to beware that there are no widowmaker trees in your area. You should also look for other possible disasters that could occur, such as rock slides, which would threaten your survival. Avoid setting up camp anywhere that would expose you to natural threats.

Wildlife is an inevitable part of the bush, and you are going to need to know how to protect yourself from them when it comes to survival. One thing to know with wildlife is that there are certain areas where they frequent, and other areas where they don't spend much time. You can tell busy areas from non-busy areas based on the amount of scat, footprints, and other tell-tale signs that wildlife has been around, such as broken brush, worn-in paths, and scratches in trees. You should also pay attention to wasps nests or hornets nests, ants nests, or anything else that could be dangerous to be situated around. Naturally, you want to stay away from these areas to avoid putting yourself in an area that is highly likely for you to become exposed to plenty of wildlife. As well, you want to consider how well your camp is set up for you to protect yourself from wildlife, such as how easy it will be to safely store your food away from camp.

Building Your Main Shelter

If you arrive at your camp late, you may only have time to build a small shelter from smaller branches and twigs nearby, as well as any tarps and groundcovers you have already brought with you. As soon as you can, however, you want to get on with making a proper shelter that you can stay in. This will require larger branches to construct a frame; then you will require items that can be used to build a roof. Dry hogweed logs, long grass or cane, spruce (not fir) needle branches or ferns, leaves, and moss are all great for constructing the top of your shelter. If you have a tarp you brought along with you, you can also use that in your roof to create a stronger layer of protection. Other materials that can be used to construct your shelter include snow, clay, bark, flat stones, and even trash.

When building your shelter, you will want to have your axe and saw handy so that you can shape your frame branches as needed, and cut things down if necessary to get them to fit into place. Your tarp, rope, and knife will also be handy to help you haul things back to camp, and a bucket and shovel will come in handy if you are using snow or clay to construct your shelter.

The easiest way to build your main shelter is to find a spot in your camp where you can naturally be sheltered. For example, if you see a dugout in the side of a rock form, a few trees huddled together, or even a hollowed-out fallen tree, you can use this as the basis for your shelter. Of course, check the safety of this space to ensure that you are not at risk of anything falling and hurting you, and to be sure that animals are not already using that shelter.

If you cannot find a natural spot with shelter, you will want to make the next best thing: an A-frame shelter. While there are many types of shelters you can build in the bush, these are simple and durable. You will build an A-frame shelter by cutting thick branches to construct an A-frame and then building your roof on top of that. For an A-frame shelter, you will want 5 Y-shaped branches and one long branch that is about 1.25 times the length of your body. You will use the Y-shape branches to prop up the larger one, which will form the peak of your roof. Avoid making your A-frame shelter too large, as they can become more at risk of being damaged by the weather if they are too big, and the branches themselves can pose a threat to your safety. Instead, keep it nice and cozy so that you are tucked safely away and so that you are able to keep yourself comfortable and warm throughout the night.

When you build your shelter, you always want to build it from the ground up. You will start with your ground cover; then, you will build your frame, then you will build out your roof. A roof should be started with a layer of branches that will provide a frame for you to add everything else to. You can use lashings and bindings to help keep everything secured and in place. Below you will find the description of some common rope techniques that you can use for camp setup. If you are using a tarp, you would add it in next. Then, you would use spruce needle branches, leaves, long grasses, or even clay to construct the rest of your roof. Make it as packed as you possibly can to avoid any leaks which would get water into your shelter.

Building Additional Shelters

In addition to your main shelter, you may want to construct additional shelters for your camp, depending on how long you will be staying. If your sleeping shelter is particularly small, you may wish to create a shaded shelter where you can sit during the day to relax and get away from the weather. This shelter can also be used as a safe place for you to prepare food and construct things for camp without bringing anything into your main sleeping shelter.

Another shelter you may want to have in your camp is a hygiene shelter. A hygiene shelter can be used for washing yourself, but it can also be used as a sort of first aid spot in your camp, providing you with a clean space to sit down and tend to any cuts, scrapes, bruises, or anything else you may have received during the day. This shelter can be small and should be kept clean at all times. It should also have a proper log or something to sit on so that the person being treated can sit safely up and away from the ground and any contaminants on the ground. Your hygiene shelter should be close to water and a fire so that you can sterilize any equipment that may need to be used during a first aid situation.

Tarp Setup

Setting up a tarp for your camp can be done in a variety of ways, depending on what you need and what size your tarp is. The terrain you are setting up in will also affect the way you set up your tarp. The four easiest ways to set up a tarp include flying a tarp, building a lean to, setting up a diamond shelter, and creating tarp tents. You will also need to consider your ground cloth to ensure that your tarp is properly insulated.

Flying a Tarp

To fly a tarp means that the edges do not touch the ground at all, creating more of a shelter over top of you. This is excellent for day shelter, or for shelter in hot areas where a tent-style shelter may be too hot to sleep in. To fly a tarp, you are going to need five lengths of rope, including one that is longer then the tarp is wide. You will set up your tarp between two trees that are relatively close together, but far enough apart that your tarp will stretch between the two of them without wrinkling or folding over. Then, you will take your longest length of rope and tie it around the trunk of one tree about 5-6 feet high, and then tie it at the same height on the other tree, pulling it taut. Next, you will toss the tarp over the taut rope so that it hangs down with half on either side. Then, you will take your four additional lengths of rope and tie them into the corners of each tarp and attach them to something nearby, such as a low stump or a sturdy branch on some nearby brush. Your tarp should look like a tent that has been raised in the air.

Tarp Tent

A tarp tent is made with a single tarp and is used to keep you sheltered from the elements. While it will not keep you warm in the cold, it will keep you away from cold winds and rains. You can then stuff the tent with insulating layers of sleeping bags, clothes, and ground cloth as needed. For your tarp tent, you will want one tarp, one tree, and one branch that has been removed from a tree. The branch should be thick enough that it will be able to stand on its own. Then, you will need string and stakes, or nearby underbrush that you can tie your tent to if stakes aren't available. You will set up your tent by first locating the center of the tarp along one side and tying that to the tree, about 4 feet high. Make it a bit lower if you have a smaller tarp, or a bit higher if you have a larger one. Then, you are going to set your branch upright a few feet away from the tree. You want it far enough away that you will have a decent shelter, but close enough that the back end of your tarp will reach the ground even once it's been draped over the branch. Next, you are going to drape the tarp over the branch and then tie or stake down the edges so that they stay neatly tucked in on the ground. If you have no stakes, you could use rocks in a pinch.

Tarp Lean-To

The tarp lean to shelter is another shelter that can easily be made using two trees that are nearby. The trees should be far enough apart that you can keep your tarp taut when tying it up. The nice thing about a lean to shelter is that it will not require the long length of rope to hold up the middle like flying a tarp will. To create your lean-to, you will simply tie one corner of the tarp to one tree and one to another. Then, with the other two corners, you can either tie them to the ground, stake them to the ground, or hold them down with heavy rocks. The result should be a tarp that is hung tightly between two trees and able to be sat under, lied under, or used to keep your gear dry.

Diamond Shelter Tarp

A diamond shelter tarp is a fly technique that allows you to fly your tarp while still getting good protection out of it. These are great for protecting you from rain or wind, and they can also be used for sleeping inside. To make your diamond shelter tarp, you will need three lengths of rope, or one length of rope and three stakes or heavy rocks to hold down the corners. The best spot to create your diamond shelter tarp will be somewhere where there is a tree you can tie it to, and where there is a low stump, branch, or tree, you can attach the other side to. You will take your long length of rope and attach it to the tree about 3-4 feet up the trunk. Then, you will tie the other end of the rope to the ground, or to a stake in the ground if you have one. You will then place the tarp over the rope diagonally so that one corner touches the tree trunk, and the opposite corner touches the ground. The other two corners will need to be staked to the ground or held in place with heavy rocks.

Ground Cloth

Ground cloth is essential for your tents as it helps insulate them and keep you warm. A proper ground cloth will keep moisture out and body heat in, effectively warming up your tent so that you do not catch a chill or endanger your precious core temperature. Ground cloth should be set corner to corner at the bottom of your tent so that you are able to keep as much heat in as possible. If you are in a hot climate and you are not using a carefully closed in shelter, you can lay a ground cloth under your sleeping bag and then sleep in, or on, the sleeping bag. Even in a drier climate, this is important as you do not want to get any moisture in your clothes. Once you get damp in the bush, it is hard to dry off, and being damp for too long can be very bad for your skin and your health.

Lashes, Bindings, and Toggles

Making lashes, bindings, and toggles are all essential skills to have if you are going to be surviving in the bush. These teach you how to make sure that your rope actually stays where you place it, effectively keeping your tools in place. The easiest techniques to learn that will also get you the furthest in the bush include square lashing, snowshoe binding, and making a basic toggle.

Square Lashing

To do square lashing, you are going to place your two items you are connecting so that they are perpendicular to each other, with a cross in the center. They will end up at a 90-degree angle once tied. For the sake of easier explaining, let's imagine you have two sticks perpendicular to one another, and you are tying them together with a square lashing. You will start by tying a knot around the bottom stick, nice and close to where the two sticks cross. Then, you will pull your rope up and over the top stick, then down and under the other side of the bottom stick, opposite of where you tied the knot. Then, you will come up around and over the top stick, opposite to the side where you went over the last time. Now, you will go under where you placed your knot. You will continue weaving over and under until you have done this three times around. Then, you will wrap all the way around the top stick next to the knot and go in the reverse direction three times. When you are done, you will tie the rope in place with a simple knot.

Simple Binding

When you are binding something together, such as one log to another, you want to make sure you do it in such a way that it is held tightly in place and won't move. This method is important if you are going to be attaching logs together so that you can form them into a roof over your shelter, or sides for your shelter. You will bind by first taking the center of a length of rope and wrapping it around a piece of wood completely so that you have one full wrap and two equal tail lengths. Then, you will wrap it completely around the piece of wood you want to attach it to before wrapping it all the way around the bottom or original piece again and coming back up either side. You will now pull it tight. If you are connecting heavier branches or logs, you will want to do this one to two more times, depending on the thickness of the branches or logs. Then, you will start wrapping them around completely but pulling them down the length of the log as you go, creating long "x" shapes across the log. When you reach the middle, you will wrap one complete circle in place. Then, you will make "x" shapes again until you reach the other end of the branch or log. There, you will make one to three tight, complete wraps again. Then, you will tie off.

Making a Toggle

Making a toggle when you are In the bush is incredibly simple. All you will do is find a sturdy material that is somewhat thin and about 2-3" wide. You want to pick something that will be steady and not break, such as a thick branch, a rock, a piece of metal, or even a piece of a larger animal's femur bone. You will then tie a piece of rope around the very center of that item. You can now insert your toggle into the grommets on your tarp to hold it up, use it to keep a rope wrapped snuggly around a tree without tying it, or even use it to hold things in your pack. If you have nothing to insert the toggle into, make a simple knot on your rope with a loop in it and insert the toggle into the loop. This will keep everything nice and tight and secure. If you are securing something heavier or larger, always use thicker, sturdier toggles to avoid having the toggle snap, and someone gets injured as a result.

Hygiene, Organization, and Protection

Keeping your camp hygienic, organized, and protected is of utmost importance. Proper hygiene will ensure that no one gets sick, organization will ensure that you can find everything you need the moment you need it, and protection will keep you safe from the elements and wildlife.

Personal hygiene can be achieved using a few methods. When you cannot safely wash in running water, consider taking a smoke bath. By lighting a fire and bathing in the smoke, the smoke kills any bacteria on your body, which effectively cleanses you. As well, the smell is less likely to attract bugs such as flies and mosquitoes. If you can find oak, hickory, birch, aspen, or poplar trees, you can take some of their bark and boil it until the water becomes dark. As soon as the water is of a manageable temperature, dip a cloth in and wash your body with the all-natural tannin body wash. For your teeth, you can use twigs from dogwood or sassafras trees, which are both useful for cleaning and excellent because they have tannic acid, which will help cleanse your teeth, much like how it helps cleanse your body. Chew up the small twigs as this is how they become fibrous and work well as toothbrushes. If you need to wash your hands, such as after dealing with an animal carcass, you will want to find a yucca plant or a yarrow plant, as both can be scrubbed across your hands to cleanse them. Avoid ingesting these plants; however, yucca, in particular, is poisonous if ingested, but it is harmless on your hands. Finally, it is critical that you keep your feet dry and clean as often as possible when it comes to living in the bush. Wear proper footgear, wash your feet regularly, dry them off completely, and keep them in clean socks and shoes as often as you possibly can. When you are navigating backwoods, your feet become exposed due to the constant walking, climbing, and navigating of rugged terrain. They can also become damp, dirty, and easily injured if you are not careful. An injured foot can quickly become infected due to ongoing exposure and use, which can lead to a dangerous and even deadly situation. Keeping your feet dry and clean is imperative at all times. If you do sustain an injury to your foot, practice maximum care in keeping it clean at all times to avoid an infection.

For camp hygiene, you want to boil and cleanse everything as soon as it is used, including camp cookware and any other tools you have been using around raw meat or other contaminants. Your clothes should be washed out as needed in a nearby stream and hung to dry in the sunlight. Whenever possible, hang things such as your bedding and worn clothes that are not quite ready to be washed yet in the sunlight. Sun kills bacteria within hours, so this is a great way to keep everything cleansed and neutralized.

Organization can be achieved in whatever way you want; however, you should have a clear system, and you should stick with that system. Keep all of your cookware in one clean spot. Keep all of your tools organized and easy to access. Keep your sleeping hut away from your eating space, and keep your firewood in an easy to access safe spot. Your food should be stored safely away from camp, yet in an easy to access spot so that if any animals do happen across it, they cannot find it, but they also cannot find you in the process.

As far as protection goes, there are many steps you can take to protect yourself. Sleeping with an axe, machete, or other similar weapons on hand is a good idea as this can help you protect yourself from any animals that may surprise you. Otherwise, never sleep in the clothes you cooked in; keep a source of light and bear spray on hand if you have any, and if you have any pets, keep them leashed and close by so they do not attract animals. Always sleep at least 100 yards away from where you store your food and do your cooking so you are not discovered if an animal discovers your food, and they will. Build your shelter in such a way that makes it challenging for anything else to get in there with you, and always keep a fire going at all hours of the day and night. Generally, fire and smoke from the fire will deter animals from bothering you. The fire you keep going near your sleep shelter should, naturally, be different from the fire you cook over.

CHAPTER 4
Building And Managing Fires

Fires are a primary tool when it comes to surviving in the woods. You are going to have at least two fires that you will need to create and maintain, though if you find yourself venturing away from camp for hunting or fishing, you may need to create additional, smaller fires on the go. Knowing how to build fires properly and safely is an essential skill for survival.

The Triangle of Fire

A fire can be started with three elements, and it can also be stopped by eliminating one of the three elements. The three elements required for fire include heat, fuel, and oxygen. In fire crafting, you want to intentionally create a safe space where you can add fuel, create heat, and maintain high oxygen levels so that your fire can thrive. You will do this by constructing a fire lay that allows ample oxygen to get in and around your fire, which allows you to place added wood (fuel) without smothering your fire, and to use the fire as needed without smothering it or hurting yourself in the process.

Anytime you build a fire in the woods, you should also be prepared to put that fire out. This way, if your fire gets out of control or needs to be eliminated for any reason, you can safely do so. The two best ways to stop a fire in the woods is to either drench it in water or smother it with dirt. Keeping a pail of water nearby can be useful to eliminate your fire, or you can shovel dirt onto it if it gets out of control to smother it.

Placing Your Fire

When you place a fire, you want to consider where the fire is going so that you can preserve the safety of your camp and maintain the benefit of the fire. Your food fire, as stated, should be kept at least 100 yards away from your sleeping arrangements. That way, if any food drippings fall into the fire or if it begins to accumulate a smell, animals will be attracted away from where you are, rather than toward where you are. Your fire for warmth, light, and protection should be built closer to your sleeping arrangements so that you can rely on it as needed. This fire should, however, be built a bit away from your sleeping arrangements so that it cannot accidentally catch your sleeping arrangements on fire and burn you in your sleep.

All fires should be built in such a way that they will be easy to contain, that they will not catch any nearby bushes and that they will not grow too high to catch the tree branches above. This way, you are not running the risk of creating a fire that is larger than you can reasonably control.

Fire Lays

The best fire lay that you can use in the woods is a teepee lay. If you are just creating a fire for warmth, you can construct a circle out of rocks on the ground and build a teepee fire inside of it. If you are looking to cook with your fire, you will want to make a smaller teepee so that your fire does not get too hot, and so that you can create a cooktop surface.

The Teepee Fire Lay

The teepee fire lay is created by taking several thick branches cut to about 2 feet long or less, depending on the height of the fire you want. Then, you will lean all of the branches up together in a cone shape, with the point toward the sky, like a teepee. You will then place kindling and fire-starting material in the center of the teepee so that you can light that part on fire. As the fire builds within the teepee, it will catch the branches on fire, effectively giving you a strong fire to keep yourself warm or to cook over.

Log Cabin Fires

A log cabin fire lay is made by taking various branches and pieces of wood that are no more than 1" thick, as this will make it easier for all of them to catch fire. You may want the wood bases to be slightly thicker though, around 1.5-2" thick so that it is more sturdy. You will then lay two sticks parallel to each other, and then run two perpendicular to them across the edges. You will go back and forth, crisscrossing your branches until they look like a pyramid. Then, you will build a similar structure around the edges of this by crisscrossing wood; only this time, you will not form them into a pyramid shape but rather keep them square. These sticks should be somewhat thicker, around 2-3" or up to 4" at the base. You won't need to build your fire too tall, maybe 4-6 levels. Then, you will light the small inner pyramid on fire and let it get going. It will then catch the larger log cabin formation outside of it on fire, giving you a nice, healthy fire to work with.

Long Log Fires

A long log fire is used if you need your fire to burn all night. This is important, especially if you are in a cooler climate or somewhere where you will need access to ongoing warmth and light. You will make your long log fire by digging a shallow depression into the ground, about 6' long and 1' wide. Then, you will build a fire that fills the length of the depression using a log cabin formation but spreading it the length of the depression. Once the fire is going, you should find that it burns down into the ground creating good hot coals and a nice roaring fire. You will then put two long logs on top of the fire, running the length of the depression. This should keep your fire running all night long.

Dakota Fire Pits

Dakota fire pits are a type of fire that is nestled into a hole that you dig into the ground. They are easily contained, provide great heat, function excellent in high wind areas, and they can help you remain stealthy if need be. A Dakota fire hole needs to be built anywhere where there is a flat surface that you can easily dig into, but where the ground is hard enough that it won't collapse when dug into. Once you have decided on your location, you need to completely clear away any vegetation from where you are going to place the fire. Then, you are going to dig a hole. A hole that is deeper will be less visible from the surface, while a hole that is wider will make a bigger fire. Pick what you need most. After you have dug out your main hole, you will need to dig a second hole on an angle, connecting into the bottom of the main hole. Do not connect the hole with your shovel, but instead dig in and connect the hole with your hand; this way, you do not accidentally collapse the earth around it. The hole should be about the size of your fist, as this is going to feed oxygen to your fire so that your fire can continue to burn. Once you have set the pit, you should start a fire in the hole using dry brush and other starting materials. Then, you can start to add larger sticks until your fire is burning consistently. Your fire is ready to go!

The Cooking Fire Lay

A simple cooking fire lay, also called a bundle fire is created by taking logs that are all about the same height and bundling them together with the cut sides both up and down, creating a flat surface on the top of them. You will hold the bundle up using bindings and rocks on either side. Then, you will light a fire under the bundle using a fire starter. As the fire begins to lick the top of your surface, you can place your pot or pan on top of the fire and cook. Note that you want to cook before the logs get too burnt as they will start to fall and could cause a dangerous situation if your pot falls into the fire and splashes water or hot food anywhere.

Starting Materials

There are many starting materials you can use when it comes to getting a fire going. If you are able to bring starting materials with you, bring cardboard, cotton swabs, dryer lint, and citrus peels or nutshells with you as these are all great fire starters. If you need to find fire-starting materials in the wild, look for pine cones, pine needles, cattails, cedar chips from splitting wood, dried grass, moss, and even small dried twigs and leaves as these are all great for starting a fire with. Avoid putting anything damp in there, such as moss or damp brush from the bottom of the forest, as these will dampen your fire and prevent any proper fire from starting.

Sourcing Wood

Sourcing wood in the woods is easy, though picking the right tree is important. There are a few things you need to consider when it comes to picking your tree. First, you want to start by looking for trees that have already died and fallen over, as they will be dry and ready to burn. If you must cut down a live tree, you will need to wait several days for it to properly dry out so that it can be burnt. Otherwise, you need to slowly add them to your fire so that the fire can dry them out first, before catching them on fire. If you must pick a live tree, pick a tree or a large branch that is not too thick so that it will dry out faster. You also want to make sure the tree is far enough away from camp that you do not risk damaging your camp if it falls over, but close enough to camp that you can haul it back.

If you are chopping back a live tree, you will cut a notch in the side facing the direction you want it to fall in. Note that it will not always fall this way, so you will still need to be careful to watch where it is going. You can create the notch by cutting into the tree at a 45-degree angle up and down so that there is a complete notch cut into the side. This notch should go no more than ¼ to 1/3 of the way into the tree to avoid making the notch so big that the tree falls while you are still cutting it. Once you have cut in your notch, you will go to the opposite side of the tree and cut straight into it. Ideally, as soon as the tree is cut through, it will fall toward the notch. You can increase this likelihood by avoiding trees that have obviously heavy branches on the side opposite of where you want it to fall, and by avoiding cutting trees on heavy wind days, especially when the wind is not blowing in a favorable direction.

After you have cut the tree, you will chop it into manageable sized logs on the spot then drag those logs back to camp. There, you can process them by cutting them down into smaller logs that are fit for burning in your fires. You should keep your log reserve full at all times to ensure that you always have fuel for your fires.

CHAPTER 5

Navigation And Tracking

Perhaps one of the scariest, yet most important skills that you need to know about when it comes to bushcrafting is navigation and tracking. Knowing how to navigate the terrain you are in, keeping track of yourself, and tracking necessary survival resources is important if you are going to survive. With that being said, it can be incredibly simple to get turned around backward in the woods and to find yourself confused with where you are, where you are going, and where you need to be. Proper navigation and tracking skills will keep you clear on where you are and easily able to navigate the terrain you are living in.

The trick with navigation is to realize that when you are stressed out and scared, it can be incredibly easy for you to forget everything and find yourself completely confused and lost. A startling sound, feeling a little too hungry, thirsty, or tired, or even an encounter with wildlife can throw you off course and have you wondering how to get back on track. For that reason, it is important that you educate yourself on navigation and tracking, practice it as often as you can, and do your best to be as meticulous as possible with navigation and tracking should you ever find yourself in a survival situation. This way, you are unlikely to find yourself permanently lost and at-risk due to exposure and a lack of protection in the woods.

Using Your Compass Properly

Knowing how to use a compass properly can seem somewhat intimidating if you have never had to do it before. Fortunately, using a compass is relatively easy and can be learned quickly. The first thing you need to know before using a compass is the different parts of the compass and what they do. Your compass has seven different parts that aid you in navigation: the baseplate, the direction of travel arrow, the compass housing, the degree dial, the magnetic needle, the orienting arrow, and the orienting lines.

The baseplate and compass housing are both parts of the casing for the compass. The baseplate is a plastic plate where the compass is embedded, where the compass housing is the plastic shell that houses the magnetized needle inside of the compass itself.

The direction of travel arrow is the arrow inside of the baseplate that points away from the arrow. The degree dial is a dial that can be twisted to display all 360 degrees of a circle. The magnetic needle points north and south. The orienting arrow is a non-magnetic arrow inside of the compass housing, and the orienting lines run parallel to the orienting arrow.

To use your compass, you will start by holding it in your flat palm and gently rotating it side to side to ensure that your magnetic arrow is properly functioning. This ensures the compass gets an accurate read, and that it is working properly. Next, you want to figure out what direction you are facing. To do this, you will turn the degree dial until the orienting arrow lines up with the north end of the magnetic arrow. Once the arrows are lined up, look at the direction of travel arrow on the baseplate, which will indicate what direction you are going. If it falls between E and S, for example, you are facing southeast.

As you look at your arrow, you will need to tell the difference between "true" north and "magnetic" north. True north refers to the point where all longitudinal lines meet up at the top of the map, also known as the north pole. Magnetic north is the tilt of the magnetic field, which is about eleven degrees different from the tilt of the earth's axis. The difference between these two measures is called "declination." This difference can cause up to 20 degrees of difference between magnetic north and true north in different terrains. You will have to account for the shift to get a truly accurate reading of your map. Note that traveling even just one degree off from what your map says can lead to you being 100 feet or 30 meters off track, which can be a major difference when traveling in the backwoods.

Correcting the declination or difference between true north and magnetic north requires you to know where the line of zero is in your area. The best way to do this is to research it ahead of time and to research the line of zero for where you are likely to find yourself in a state of survival. This way, you can be sure that you have true north. This will matter most when you find yourself following someone else's map, as any official map will be made using true north, not magnetic north for that area.

When you are ready to begin traveling, you need to start by finding your bearings. Twist the dial until the orienting arrow, and the north end of the magnetic arrow is aligned, then pay attention to where you are now. If you have a true map you are following, adjust your dial for the declination in your area. Next, you need to identify the exact direction you need to be going, and then you need to hold your compass up to help ensure that you are walking in that direction the entire time. If you are unable to hold your compass up for extended periods of time, you can do what is called "leapfrogging." Leapfrogging means that you identify your intended direction, identify an object in the distance that exactly aligns with that direction, and walk there until you reach that location. Then, you take out your compass and check for your next directional point. Keep doing this until you get where you need to go.

When you have a map that has already been created, either by you or someone else, you can use that map to help you find your direction of travel and to help you find your bearings. To do this, place your map on a horizontal surface and lay your compass over the directional arrow points on the map so you can identify true north. Then, slide your compass until it's edge crosses over your current location with the orienting arrow still pointing north. Draw a line along the edge at your current position. Taking your bearing from the map this way will require you to then identify the exact point where you want to end up. Next, use the edge of your compass to create a line between where you are and where you want to go. Now, rotate your degree dial so that the orienting arrow points toward true north, and identify exactly what direction you need to head in order to get where you are going based on the direction of your compass. Simply follow that direction until you reach your intended point, as this will give you a new bearing to help you navigate your terrain with.

Following a Map

Ideally, you want to gather a printed map (or two) of the location you will be living in so that you know exactly where everything is. This will make locating a campsite, discovering water, and learning the terrain much faster. You can often find specific survival maps online for the location where you expect you will be surviving in when you leave an urban environment. When it comes to following a map, especially a detailed map of the environment you are in, there are a few things you need to know to help you follow that map.

Topographic maps, or maps of back wood locations, will have details that allow you to know what type of terrain is being represented on the map, and what distances are being represented on the map. The scale will generally be shown in miles and will show you how much of the map represents a certain amount of miles. For example, one inch on the map may represent 2 miles in real life. If your terrain has mountains in it, there will be another scale that shows you how to identify the heights of those mountains. Mountains are represented by round lines that encompass the entirety of the mountain itself, and every fifth line is thicker and has an actual number identifying the height of that part of the terrain. If the circles represented on your map are notched all the way around, this means you are looking at a depression or a valley, rather than a mountain.

Other terrains, including peaks, ridgelines, cliffs, peaks, valleys, saddles, places with sparse vegetation, and spaces with dense vegetation, will also be visible on your map. Each map will come with a legend that lets you know what each color means and what each symbol on the map means, effectively helping you determine what the terrain around you looks like.

Maps have five colors on them, including brown, green, blue, black, and red. Brown represents contour lines, which indicate elevation. Green represents vegetation. Blue represents water sources. Black represents man-made objects or structures. Red represents major roadways. White represents "nothing." For example, if you see a white space with some green splashed within it, this means the area has sparse vegetation, and nothing significant around it, as well as no significant inclination or sloping.

When you are traveling long distances, you will want to identify the different points where you will be passing through as you travel so that you can create milestones in your path. This way, you can aim toward each milestone and practice leapfrogging to help you get there. Then, you can pull out your map and find your next location to head toward. In due time, you will find yourself exactly where you need to be.

The Five Navigation Methods You Need

As you travel, there are five navigation methods that will help you feel confident that you are exactly where you need to be, and that you are safe. These methods will also help you maintain your bearings and successfully navigate your way to your destination. They include handrails, backstops, baselines, aiming off, and panic azimuths.

Handrails are a form of navigation method whereby you use a certain feature or item to create a guide that takes you where you want to go. Once you navigate your way to a handrail, you simply need to follow it, and you can trust that it will take you where you need to go. Handrails can either be a certain element on your map, or they can be something you create yourself. For example, if you are in an area that has a body of water, you may use a certain length of the body of water as a handrail to guide you toward where you are going. As long as you stay near the water for that amount of time, you know you are where you need to be. You will also easily be able to find yourself again. Making your own handrail can be done by having a particular marker that you use to track out a certain trail or area where you will be heading to frequently, such as a popular place for hanging snares or the area where you will be cooking your food. You can make your own markers by marking trees or branches with certain marks, by tying something around multiple trees or branches along the way, or by otherwise marking your trail. This way, you know exactly where to go every single time.

Backstops are landmarks you hit that you will not cross at any given time. They are important as they prevent you from traveling too far. If you hit a backstop, you know you need to stop and turn around. You should define backstops on all four sides of your camping area, and define backstops anytime you are leaving camp to go somewhere. Even if you are not intending on going far, backstops will help.

Baselines are geographic boundaries that are designed to keep you in certain areas. While your backstop is designed to prevent you from traveling out of bounds, your baseline can help you identify where you are and how to get where you are going. A great example of a baseline would be a main road or a major trail traveling along the length of your camp. These would be fairly easy to stumble across and, once you were on them, you would have a good idea of where you are and where you need to go from there to get back to where you need to be.

Aiming off is a method that allows you to deliberately set yourself on a course that is off to one side of your destination. For example, let's say where you need to go is exactly northwest of where you are, you would purposefully go a little further north. The reason for aiming off is that it allows you to get exactly where you need to go every single time by knowing exactly where your destination is from where you have arrived. Let's say that you are going out to set traps, and there is a cliff as a backstop for your trip. If you tried to aim directly for where you have set your traps, you might be a few degrees off and then miss your traps. At this point, you would know whether to go left or right because you would not know whether you had gone a little too far to the right or to the left when you were traveling to find your traps. If, however, you had purposefully aimed off to the right, you would know that no matter how off you may have been, all you have to do is turn left and walk along the cliff to find your traps. Purposefully aiming off a little to the wrong direction ensures that once you reach that destination, you know exactly which way to go to get to your actual destination, and it is a lot easier to get there because now you are much closer. In other words, it makes it easier for you to keep your bearings.

Panic azimuths are basically backup plans when you are traveling, and they are the easiest way to find yourself when you are lost. A panic azimuth should be planned out before you leave, and it should be used anytime you find yourself either lost or dealing with a problem that requires you to abort your mission in the bush. Essentially, you are going to pick a specific direction that you will walk in order to help yourself become found again. For example, let's say your cooking camp is 100 yards southeast of your sleeping camp. Perhaps you set off to get there but were a few degrees off and so now you cannot find your cooking camp. At this point, you would either decide to go only south or only east until you reach a familiar landmark that helps you find yourself. Pick one based on what is easiest in your terrain. For example, if south of your cooking area, there is a nearby body of water, then only go south until you reach that body of water. At that point, you will have a general idea as to where you are and how to get back to camp from there.

Determining Distance When Traveling

Maps always define how to get somewhere based on the number of miles or number of kilometers traveled. When you have an actual navigation system on you, it is easy to identify how far you have traveled. However, in the backwoods, digital navigation systems are unavailable, so you are going to need to know how to measure how far you have traveled to ensure that you do not go too far, or not reach quite far enough. Pedometers, or step counters, are a great way to keep track of yourself in the bush. With a pedometer, the device counts the number of steps you take. You should make sure your pedometer is well calibrated in advance to avoid having an ill calibrated pedometer throwing you off course. It takes roughly 2,000 steps for an adult to walk one mile, so you will need to calculate your course based on that. For example, if you know you need to go 1.5 miles east before turning south, you will need to go roughly 3,000 steps east before turning south. Be sure to keep track of your pedometer to avoid getting lost.

Finding Yourself When You're Lost

Panic azimuths are the fastest and easiest way to find yourself when you are lost in a bush. If, however, you find yourself still lost, there are two options you can take to help you find yourself. The first option is to climb to the highest ground you can reach and look around to see where you are. This should help you get an idea of where you need to go in order to find yourself. The other option is to follow the land or keep walking until you find a body of water and then follow the body of water until you reach someplace familiar. If you do not seem to find your way back to camp or civilization, be sure to look out for evidence of human existence. A trailblazer, tire tracks, previous campfires, and other such things are great evidence that humans have been around, and if you follow these signs, you should be able to find your way out in no time. Finally, you can use the sun as a compass if you need to. The sun rises in the east and sets in the west, so as long as you know whether it is morning or afternoon, you can use the sun to help guide you. If it is morning, the sun will be in the eastern sky, while if it is afternoon, it will be in the western sky. If it is dead ahead, this means it is noon. Wait about an hour or so, and the sun will move toward the west, and you will be able to use it to guide your way back to camp again.

CHAPTER 6

Securing And Storing Food And Water

After you have secured shelter and fire, which will protect your core temperature, you need to start focusing on securing yourself food and water. Water should count as your first order of business, as you can only live for 3 days without water, whereas you can live for up to 3 weeks without food. With that being said, the longer you go without either, the weaker you will become, and the harder it will be for you to get any.

If you arrive at your campsite in the late afternoon, your only order of business should be to secure some water. If you arrive in the evening or later, you should wait until morning and do with whatever you have in your pack until then. You will last one night, even if you are beginning to feel uncomfortable. As soon as morning comes, you should fetch yourself some water and then prepare to get yourself some food. Even if you were able to bring food along with you and you are able to eat a decent breakfast, you should be on the hunt for food from day one. It can take a bit to get the hang of catching game, even if you have done it in the past, as you will have to be able to track the animals and set traps to catch them. That can take time. The sooner you get started, the sooner you will have a steady supply of food to keep you going.

Purifying and Storing Water

If you were able to prepare properly for a survival setting, you should have a bottle or a water filter that allows you to filter water right out of the water source. With that being said, even after the water has been filtered, you should still boil it to sterilize it from any potential bacteria that may have gotten through. It is always better to air on the side of caution, as water can contain harmful bacteria and parasites that can be dangerous to your health.

If you do not have a filter on hand, you can make a natural one using things you find in nature, as well as a shirt or a large piece of fabric. You will create your filter by placing your fabric over the top of a pot so that it caves in, somewhat like a bowl. Fix it in place, so it doesn't move. Then, you will add charcoal from the fire pit, dirt, sand, grass, and gravel on top of it. Next, you will pour your water through the homemade filter until it reaches the pot. Then, you will boil it to eliminate any further contaminants. While this is not the ideal solution, it will give you the best chance of being able to purify your water so that you are far less likely to fall ill from drinking it. You should keep your canteens full at all times, so you will likely need to fetch, filter, and boil water every day or every other day. Always do it before you completely run out, as you will want the boiling water to have plenty of time to cool down before you consume it. As well, make sure you cover the boiled water properly to avoid having any contaminants falling in after you have already cleaned it out.

Preparing to Trap Animals

Protein is essential in the bush, as you are using large amounts of energy. Protein is a slower burning fuel, so to speak, making it perfect for the type of energy you need for survival. You can source protein using traps. Trapping animals in the bush is the easiest way to source animals when you are without typical hunting tools like guns, bows, and arrows. If you do happen to have any of the latter on hand, though, you could use them to harvest larger mammals. With that being said, larger mammals are not ideal in the bush as you end up with more meat than you can reasonably eat or store, and that becomes a large threat as you are more likely to attract hungry animals who could attack you in the process of trying to steal your meat. If you do manage to ward off animals, you are still at risk of the meat spoiling before you can consume it all. And, lastly, you want to save your munitions for protection, just in case an animal comes up, and you are unable to reasonably escape or protect yourself without your weapons.

Trapping animals is relatively simple. All you need is an idea of where animals tend to spend most of their time, bait, and a properly made and set trap to help you capture the animals. Below, you will find everything you need to locate animals and trap them safely and as humanely as possible.

Signs for Finding Game

Animal signs are the key to successful trapping as these indicate that there are clearly animals present to be trapped. It can take some practice to find animal signs, as animals are rather good at hiding their tracks to avoid being hunted by other wildlife. Even so, you can still find them if you pay close attention. The signs of an animal being present include scat, fur, burrows, sounds, hordes of food, runways or rub marks, and animal tracks or claw marks.

Scat is often found along an animal's typical trail since wild animals are not known for seeking out specific areas to go to the bathroom. Fresh animal droppings will be shiny and soft, while any scat that has been out for a while will be dry and crumbly. You can identify the animal based on the size and shape. When you are trapping animals for food, you will want to find animals with scat that is relatively small, as this will indicate that you are following the track of a rabbit, a hare, or something of similar size and shape.

Fur is something that is commonly found in spring and fall, as animals tend to shed and grow new coats around this time of year. Even so, animals will shed mildly throughout most of the year, so you may find tufts of fur scattered around the area when you are tracking an animal. If you see fur in the area, it is a good sign that an animal has been present.

Burrows are good to look for, particularly when you are hunting for survival as they indicate the presence of a small or medium animal being present. You can also look for nests if you are looking to trap birds, as these indicate that birds are around. Note, however, that nests may be abandoned outside of breeding season in the spring and early summer, so nests alone may not be a strong enough indicator that birds are actively present.

Runways and rub marks are a good indicator that animals are present. Runways are trails that have been used so frequently that they are well worn in by the animal that is using them. If you were to follow a runway long enough, it is likely that you would eventually come across an animal or, at the very least, their home. Rub marks are from animals rubbing against things like trees, branches, or bushes. Larger mammals like deer, moose, bear, and other similar animals will leave rub marks from their antlers or claws higher up on trees. Be sure to watch for these, as moose and bear, in particular, can be very dangerous to come across so you will want to avoid being in these areas too much without some form of protection.

If you sit still and quiet long enough, you may begin to hear animals nearby, or even spot one if you are lucky. Sounds and spotting animals are surefire ways of knowing that an animal is, without a doubt, present.

Bait for Trapping

The type of bait you will use for animal traps depends on what type of animal you are targeting. For many rodents, their primary food source is either vegetation, or smaller meat sources. Leaving a small bite of fresh meat may seem like a great way to bait your trap. However, you are far more likely to attract larger animals with the scent, too, which can destroy your trap and possibly invite larger predators into the area, which will then compete for your food. Instead of using meat, find fresh berries, nuts, seeds, and other foraging foods and place them in a small pile like a buffet near your trap. This will encourage rodents to come without alerting larger predators to the idea of food being in the area.

The Components of a Trap

Every trap needs an anchor that will keep it in place, and an element that will actually trap the animal. The most simple traps to set are snares, and they are made by having snare wire, a slip knot, and a place to secure your snare so that an animal is not able to take off after getting caught. Another thing you need to be aware of is something that you yourself may not be able to detect, but that the animal you are attempting to trap will. That is, your scent. Unlike humans, animals have an additional capacity to smell heavy moisture-borne molecules and pheromones. Washing your hands or rubbing your hands on your body or each other before touching your trap can contaminate it with your small. Likewise, touching the trap too much can do the same. You want to minimize your contact with the snare and, if possible, wear gloves to prevent yourself from touching it. As well, do not wash your hands before you create and set snares, instead let them, and yourself, develop a natural odor first. This way, you are less likely to warn an animal that a trap is present. Finally, as one last word of caution, never, ever touch the noose part of a trap after it has been set. A properly set trap *will* seal, quickly, and cut severely cut you or even cut one of your digits off. Both of these are not ideal as they can pose an even higher threat in the wild as they already would in normal, everyday life.

Grave's Bait Triggered Snare

A graves bait triggered snare is the easiest snare to set, and it encourages animals to come into the snare itself, making you more likely to be able to trap animals this way. Building a grave's bait triggered snare requires you to have a spring pole, a forked stake, a pencil-diameter toggle stick, a snare line with an attached trigger line, a bait stick, and bait.

To set one, you will tie a snare line to the end of a spring pole, which is a long tree branch that can easily be bent without breaking. You can find a spring pole fresh off of any tree, as long as they are fairly thin and fresh they should bend easily. You will want to have one end of the pole firmly planted in the ground where it will stay put. Then, you will bend the other end of the spring pole over until it touches the ground, then mark that spot. Next, you will drive the forked stake into the ground in that exact spot, which will be used to keep the snare nice and open so that an animal will easily fit through it. If your snare collapses at all, it will be unlikely to catch anything. Next, you are going to tie your toggle to the end of the trigger line on your trap. Then, you will run the toggle under the fork on the stake, keeping it parallel to the ground and at a right angle to the stake. Your baited trigger stick should be set at the end of the toggle, which will set the trap. Now, you just need to go away and wait for it to trap something!

Fixed Snare

Fixed loop snares are made from solid wires or braided steel cables which offer strength, flexibility, and rigidity. These traps can only be used once, as once the animal has been taught, they will typically destroy the snare from kicking and attempting to break free. Aside from this fact, these snares are the fastest and easiest to create and set.

You will set your snare using a twig that is around 1/8" to 3/16" diameter. It should be breakable. You will wind one end of your wire around the twig three times then twist the twig in circles, causing the wire to twist closed. Next, you will break the twig off, which will reveal a circle left behind. Feed the other end of the wire through that circle, and you are left with a noose. These snares work best over burrows or runways, though they can also be used on spring poles to catch game.

Drowning Snare

A drowning snare is simple and can help you quickly put any animal out of its misery, often much faster than any of the other traps will. To successfully set a drowning snare, you will require a heavy rock, a stick that floats, a snare line with a noose made into it, and a stick to prop up the rock.

You will want to find a steep-banked waterway that animals frequently use to access water. Then, tie the snare line to the rock, leaving a length of snare line available for you to tie to a float stick. Next, you will set the nose in a runway or slide that heads straight to the water, and you will prop the rock up so that it will fall (easily) once the snare is activated. The minute the snare is activated, the rock should fall into the water, dragging the animal in behind it and drowning them. The float stick will show you where the animal is so that you can quickly grab it. This type of trap is great in cold water conditions as it preserves the animal and keeps it safe from scavengers.

Squirrel Pole Snare

A squirrel pole snare can be set using a 4' to 6' pole that is around the diameter of your arm. You will cover it in fixed snares and then prop it against a tree that has signs of squirrels frequenting that tree. Squirrels love shortcuts, so one will be likely to run up or down the pole, effectively catching themselves in the snare. Be sure to set several snares on one pole to maximize your chances of catching one.

Paiute Deadfall

A Paiute deadfall is set with the intention of delivering a killing blow to the back of a small mammals head with thanks to a fairly large rock. These traps were originally made by Native American hunters and trappers, and they work incredibly well. To hunt a prairie dog or a rat, you will need an 8" long "Y" shaped stick. You will also need a straight stick that is 9" and a bit thicker than a pencil, and a 2" stick that is thinner than a pencil. A slender bait stick will be needed, too. The bait stick should be about 12" and half the diameter of a pencil. Lastly, you will need about 8" of string, bait, and a flat rock that is around 5-10 pounds.

You will start by taking the 9" straight stick and tying a string to one end of it. Then, you will tie the other end around the 2" toggle. You will want to either wipe or skewer the bait on one end of the 12" bait stick. Now, you are going to stand the "Y" shaped stick up by the edge of the rock, with the "Y" part upright. The end of the 9" stick that does not have a string attached should be placed in the fork of the "Y" shaped stick, with only 1" of it toward the rock itself. Now, you are going to lift the edge of the rock up and prop it on the 1" piece of the 9" stick. Now, you are going to wrap the toggle halfway around the post, doing a 180-degree turn. You should be able to hold the rock up by the toggle itself, without actually having to hold the rock in place. Now, you're going to place the baited end of the 12" bait stick between the bottom of the stone and the toggle. As soon as the animal taps the 12" bait stick, the toggle will release, and the rock will drop on them, effectively delivering a killing blow.

Making a Small Trapping Kit for Your Pack

Having a trapping kit on hand when you are going into the bush at any time is important, as you never know when you may need to trap an animal. With that being said, you should educate yourself on trapping laws in your area beforehand, as certain areas have rendered trapping, or certain varieties of trapping, illegal.

Creating a trapping kit requires just three easy steps, and it can be kept in your pack or in your survival jacket whenever you are away from camp. Having a trapping kit ensures that you have everything you need to set traps, which will protect you in a survival setting. The first step to making a trapping kit is to add your snares. Keep braided steel cable, cord, and wire in your trapping kit so that you have everything you need for trapping. Ideally, you should keep an assortment of thicknesses and lengths so that you can trap anything at any size that you may need to in the bush.

Next, you are going to need some bait. MRE pouches of peanut butter last years in a survival kit and work perfectly for luring small animals such as rodents in your traps. A small tin of sardines can be useful, too, as you can rub a bait stick in the sardines and place it in your snare.

Lastly, you need something to help you eliminate your scent from the trap as animals will smell you and avoid your trap altogether if they catch your scent. De-scenting spray can be found in most hunting and fishing stores, and they work to help eliminate the scent off of traps. Powdered charcoal works, too, as you can rub your hands in it and then set your traps, as charcoal will absorb odors and cover your scent. Finally, an unscented trash bag or other similar things could be used as they will provide a complete barrier between your hands and the trap.

Fishing With Improvised Rods

If you find yourself having to fish when you are in the wild, the best way to do so is through making an improvised rod. Taking a simple stick about two or three finger widths wide and around 4' to 5' long will work perfectly. You will want to keep it relatively short and thick, as this ensures that the end will not snap off in the process. You can then attach a fishing line to the end of the stick, and attach a small hook with bait on the other end. A worm or a small bug works perfectly when baiting fish.

You will want to find an area where fish tend to congregate. Pools of water next to larger moving bodies of water are great, as they tend to accumulate a large amount of fish who are taking a rest from swimming. Go in the early morning or later day, as this is when you are likely to find the most fish gathered. Then, drop your line in and flick it above the surface of the water a few times to garner interest. Let it hang for a few seconds before doing it again. If nothing happens, let the line sink into the water a little bit and drag it around to make your bait act like a real bug. This will do wonders in attracting the attention of fish.

CHAPTER 7

Processing Game Meat

Once you have caught an animal to eat, you are going to need to know how to process it so that you can safely consume it. Processing game meat properly is imperative, as it allows you to achieve two things. First, properly processing your meat prevents you from damaging the meat before you even get a chance to eat it. Organs such as the stomach, the bladder, and the anus contain substances that will destroy the meat. Anything that comes out of the inside of the stomach, bladder, or anus will contaminate the meat to the point where it is no longer safely consumable by humans. You must be cautious when processing meat to avoid damaging the organs and destroying your meat in the process. Secondly, you need to process it properly so that you can cook it thoroughly to avoid catching any bacteria, viruses, or parasites that an animal may have had. You also need to practice regular, every-day hygiene when processing and eating game by washing your hands thoroughly and keeping yourself clean so that you do not spread bacteria, viruses, or parasites through contaminated hands or cookware.

Small Mammals

Small mammals like rats, prairie dogs, and squirrels all need to be butchered carefully as they are well-known for carrying highly infectious diseases. Squirrels, for example, still carry the black plague even though it has been eradicated from humans. Exercising caution when preparing these animals ensures that they are properly prepared for eating and that they are able to be cooked thoroughly to avoid falling ill from consuming their meat.

The first step in processing small mammals is to make a small incision in the belly of the animal. Take care just to cut through the skin, and not through the meat itself, to avoid puncturing the organs. Next, you will make a cut all the way around the torso, just under the skin. Again, you do not want to cut the meat; you are just cutting through the skin. Now, you are going to work your fingers under the skin on the side where the backbone is, and then you will pull the skin off, pulling the top half over the head and the bottom half over the bottom of the animal. All the meat should still be intact at this point. Now, you will cut the back legs, neck, and tail, then remove them all from the animal.

Now, you will use your game shears to cut into the anus, up through the pelvis, and all the way into the neck. With two fingers, you will open the cut you have made and grab the heart, lungs, and esophagus. Pull them gently yet firmly down toward the tail, which will cause them all to easily fall out of the body cavity, leaving you with a clean inner cavity. Lastly, you will rinse the animal and place it in a bag or a bucket to carry it back to camp with you.

Medium Mammals

Medium size mammals are a little easier to butcher because they are larger, which means they're not quite as finicky. You will still need to be careful with your blade to avoid destroying your meat. With that being said, you will receive more cuts from your meat because there is more meat to cut in the first place. While small mammals like rodents are generally kept as one single piece of meat, medium mammals will be cut into different portions, creating multiple pieces of meat to be cooked and consumed.

The following explanation for how to butcher a medium mammal will be written for a hare specifically, but it can be used on any medium mammal such as a bobcat, a fox, an otter, or any other similarly sized animal.

You will start by making something for you to hang the animal from. In the bush, you could simply tie two lengths of rope tightly around the back legs of the mammal and then hang them from a low hanging branch where it is easy for you to reach the entirety of the animal for processing it.

Once the animal is hung, you will place a bucket under it and then use game shears to cut off the head and the two front feet. Wait until the animal completely bleeds out into the bucket below before moving on to the next step. Once your animal has completely bled out, you will make two incisions around the ankles on the back legs. These incisions should only go deep enough to cut into the pelt, but not the meat, and should completely detach the leg skin from the foot skin. Facing the back of the animal, or where the animal's spine is, you will take your knife and cut another incision from the inner part of the incision on the ankle down above the tail, leaving the tail and the anus intact. You will now do this again on the other leg. There should be a "V" shaped tuft of fur remaining over the tail. Go around to the stomach side of the animal and do the same thing, cutting a "V" shape out around the genitalia. Now, because you have clipped off the front feet and head, you should be able to use your hands to firmly, yet gently tug the entire pelt right off the animal, pulling down toward the ground. If you will be surviving for a while, you will want to cut down either side of the pelt so that you have two pelts: one side from the stomach, and one side from the back. Then, you will hang it taut between several branches, away from where any animals could reach it, to help it dry out. These can be used to help warm up a cold tent, to insulate your clothes and keep you warm, or for any other number of purposes in a survival camp.

With the pelt off the animal, you will now cut the two front legs off and put them in your "keep" bucket, not the blood bucket. You will need to use a sharp knife to hack through the joint, as you will not necessarily be cutting through the bones but rather breaking them apart so that you can rip the leg off while simultaneously cutting the meat from the shoulder so that you end up with two leg pieces.

Now, you will go to the backside of the animal and run your blade down one length of the spine, cutting as deep as the ribs. Then, you will do it again on the other side. When you insert your hand here and pull the meat away from the backbone, you should see spaces where you can cut the meat away from the animal altogether. Make those cuts and place those in your keep bucket with the front legs and any organs you may have harvested.

Next, from the stomach side of the animal, you will make a small 1" incision in the stomach of the animal. Then, you will insert your hands into the stomach incision and gently press the organs back and pull the skin forward. Very carefully cut the skin all the way down to the clavicle or the shoulder bone. Be careful not to damage any of the organs in the process, or else the meat will become useless. Once the stomach has been opened, carefully use your hand to pull all of the organs outside of the incision. You may want to harvest the heart, kidneys, and liver to consume as organ meat. However, it is not necessary. Do be aware that more parasites will be likely to live inside of organ meats, so if you choose to consume them, they will need to be cooked until they are well-done to thoroughly kill off any bacteria, viruses, or parasites.

Lastly, you want to cut off the two back legs of the animal by cutting close to the tail and straight down, and then over. Again, you will need to use the knife to help dislodge the joint and cut the meat at the same time. The backbone, tail, and bone pieces of the animal can then be discarded, and the legs can be kept. Rinse the meat off and then cook it!

If you are in a serious survival situation, bones from medium mammals can be used as tools. So, you may want to take the entire carcass back to camp and boil the skeleton until the meat is falling off. Then, remove the skeleton from the water, and when it is cool enough, pull all of the meat off. You will want to boil the clean bones one more time to neutralize any bacteria. Store them somewhere where you can easily access them. They can be turned into toggles, used to stake things down, sharpened to help spear fish out of the water, and even carved into sewing needles in a pinch.

Birds

Harvesting birds is entirely different from mammals because you have to remove the feathers. While pelts can be removed easily and usually in one fell swoop, feathers must be removed one at a time. The easiest way to pluck a bird is to start by cutting the wing of the bird off at the "elbow" joint in the wing, or the joint further down from the shoulder. This part of the wing is not meaty and is therefore not worth keeping.

Next, you will boil a large pot of water that is big enough for you to completely dunk the bird into the water. Then, holding the feet, you will dunk the bird in the water and hold it there for one and a half minutes. It is important to submerge the bird using oven-safe mitts and to pull it back out using tongs, as you do not want to burn yourself on hot water or steam. Once the minute and a half has gone by, you will pull the bird back out and lay it on a flat surface. Then, you will remove the feathers from the tail up to the head. They should easily fall right out at this point.

Now, you are going to cut through the skin at the point of the breast bone and cut straight along the center of the breastbone toward the center of the legs. You can pull the two pieces of skin outward, away from each other, so that they tug right off the meat. If they are stubborn, use your knife to separate the skin from the meat.

Flip the bird over onto its stomach and fold the wings all the way out and up. Cut behind each shoulder blade down to the bottom of the wing, and then cut off the feet. With birds, you will want to make a few incisions around the knee joint and then bend it back and forth until it breaks off. Now, you're going to cut and pull the skin and fat off from around the legs and thighs.

Finally, you want to cut off the wings completely and remove the remaining skin. Then, you will cut off the bird's back legs running along the side of the bird and into the fold of the thigh and down toward the tail space. Then, you will make cuts between the body and throat, coming to a "V" shape from either side of the throat. This will allow you to pull the neck of the bird out and any inner organs out, too. Lastly, you will carefully make an incision down the back from the neck incision until you reach the gut pouch. Then, you will pull it out and rip it free. Immediately dispose of the gut tract. Rinse your bird and cook it up!

Fish

Fish are probably the easiest to process at camp. Once you catch one, you will use the side of your blade to descale the fish. Run the side of your blade across the fish, dragging it side to side and always pulling away from the blade itself, until all of the scales have been removed. Then, remove the fins, the head all the way back to the gills, and the tail. Next, you will hold your knife horizontally and insert it into the fish by the tail end and carefully cut up about halfway through the fish and drag your blade toward the head, creating a horizontal incision along the length of the fishes belly. You will then carefully open the fish, reach in, and remove its entire innards. Wash the fish and prepare to cook it!

Reptiles and Amphibians

Reptiles and amphibians are common in some areas, and eating them is a good way of getting protein into your system. Reptiles and amphibians will differ in how they are processed based on whether or not they have legs. If they do have legs, but they are incredibly small, such as on a skink, you will more or less follow the same method for processing a reptile without legs, like a snake. You will simply cut the legs off as they are too small to eat anyway.

You will start to butcher an amphibian by cutting off all of its feet. Then, you will flip the amphibian over and use your game shears to cut through the skin of the amphibian. Start just above the thigh on one of the back legs and cut across the belly toward the other thigh. This part can be tough as amphibians tend to have very thick, tough skin, so be careful not to cut your hands in the process. With the incision started, go ahead and continue it around the back of the amphibian. Then, insert your fingers in through the incision and tug the skin off the rump and the top of the amphibian. Now, you will chop the legs off at the waist, keeping the two legs attached to each other. Then, you will chop one more time to separate the legs from the amphibian. While you could attempt to process the upper half of the amphibian, there will be a lot of organs in there, which makes it challenging and results in you not getting much meat out of it. So, just eat the legs. Be sure to rinse them and prepare them for cooking once you are done.

Snakes should be hung by the tail. Then, you should cut their heads off and give them time to bleed out. Then, you will use a sharp knife and make an incision on the belly part starting at the head and splitting the snake all the way back to the tail. Now, you will separate the skin from the meat, starting at the head side, and peel up toward where the snake has been tied. Discard the skin and use a pair of game shears and your hands to carefully remove and discard the innards. Now, cut off the tail end. Your snake is ready to be cooked.

Cooking Your Meat

Cooking meat in the bush always needs to be done properly to avoid making yourself sick. The easiest way to cook your meat is to cook it over a campfire like you are cooking over a stove. You can do this by putting your meat into one of your cooking pots or pans and cooking it until it is extremely well done all the way through. Ideally, you want to cook it until it is *more* done than you would at home since you will not have a meat thermometer handy to help you check for doneness. Further, many of the animals you may catch may not be able to be checked for doneness since they are not often standard to eat. It is likely that the outside of your meat will look charred and burnt, but that is exactly what you want, so long as your meat was cooked over fairly low temperatures. You can achieve the perfect temperature for cooking meat this way by cooking it over the embers of a low burning fire, which ensures that it is hot but not *too* hot.

Another way you can cook meat over the fire is by skewering it onto the end of a stick. Start by holding the stick in the heat near the fire for a few minutes to sterilize it. Then, skewer the meat onto the end of the stick and hold the meat down low into the edge of the base of the fire where the embers are burning it. Rotate it regularly and cook it until it is crispy and well-cooked all the way through. Again, look for charred edges and what would normally be considered "overcooked" to ensure that any possible contaminants are killed off, and you are safe to consume the meat.

Preserving Meat

Trapping more meat than you need for a single meal is a great way to make sure that you are able to have plenty to eat for a while, but then comes the question of how to preserve it. You need to be able to safely preserve *and* store your meat in a way where it will be cooked enough to keep you from getting sick and where it will not attract animals to your camp and put you in harms' way. Once you begin preserving meat, it is important that you know that you need to exercise extra caution when going back to the place where you have stored your meat to avoid being ambushed by a predator while you are trying to fetch your meat.

Drying

Before you can preserve your meat, you need to keep it cool, keep it clean and keep it dry. Let's say you have just caught something; you are going to want to process it and clean it in cool water as quickly as possible, which will help you keep that meat cool and ready to be cooked or preserved when the time comes. If you gather meat from your traps and it is particularly hot out, you should consider processing your meat near the trap so that you can get the pelt and guts separated. Then, you can clean the meat in a cool stream or in cool water. If it is particularly hot out, consider carrying two containers to move your meat in a smaller bucket, and a larger one. Fill the larger one with a bit of cool water, then place the smaller one inside of it and put your meat in there. This will weigh more to carry around, but it will also keep your meat cooler and prevent it from spoiling before you can either cook or preserve it.

If you are going to dry meat for preservation, the quickest way to do so is to use the sun as your tool. Slice your meat into thin strips, taking care not to leave any thick areas on the strips as thicker areas will take longer to dry and could develop harmful bacteria before try are dried.

You also need to cut away any fat as it will not dry properly. Then, you need to cool, clean, and dry the surface of the meat using the aforementioned methods. Then, you will hang the meat high in a tree or from another structure that will be challenging for any wildlife to get it. The meat should be high enough above the ground that no one can stand up and reach it and low enough from the branch that no one can reach down from the top of the branch and get it. It should also be kept in the sunlight so that the sun can quickly dry everything out.

Drying your meat this way will keep your meat good for 1-2 months. With that being said, always tear a piece of meat in half, first, to ensure there is no moisture inside before you eat it.

Smoking

Smoking meat changes the surface of the meat to one that is more acidic, which will effectively kill off any bacteria in the meat and any bacteria that try to contaminate the meat. This works the same way that using smoke to cleanse yourself works. As well, the taste of smoked meat is quite delicious for many.

It is important to note that smoking is not the same as cooking. You are bathing the meat in smoke, not warming it up from the fire, and that dries it out and preserves it. It is important to choose a good hardwood when smoking your meat, such as hickory, cherry, maple, applewood, or oak. Softwoods like pine or spruce will have way too much resin in them, and they will damage the quality of flavor in your meat.

The best wood for smoking is dry wood or dead wood that has already fallen from the tree or been cut off and sitting to dry for weeks. Fresh cut wood will produce wet smoke, which will not work well in curing your meat.

To cure your meat with smoke, you will start by slicing it thin. Then, you will make a diamond shelter tarp lay, while using another tarp to cover the "entrance" into your tarp "hut." You want to build your diamond shelter tarp lay on top of a small hill, with the "entrance" facing down the hill rather than up. Then, you will dig a fire pit into the ground near the entrance of the tarp, but not at the entrance of the tarp, to avoid catching the tarp on fire. Next, you will light the fire and use rocks to block half of the fire that is away from the makeshift smokehouse so that the smoke can only blow toward the tarp. You will then prop the entrance of the tarp partially open where all of the smoke is billowing from so that the smoke billows into the makeshift smokehouse. It should take you about a day to get a week or so worth of meat preserved this way, though if you are able to smoke for 2 straight days, you should have enough for a month. The meat is done when it is completely dried all the way through from the smoke.

Storing Your Preserved Meat

Anytime you preserve meat, you need to store it properly and safely. Preserved meat should be stored 100 yards away from your cook site, and your campsite. You can easily form a triangle shape with 100 yards between each corner of the triangle. This will keep animals away from your cook site and ensure that your cookware is unlikely to become bothered.

Store your meat in a double or even triple wrapped bag with fabric and tarp, and if you can, layer charcoal from the campfire between two of the layers to attempt to mask some of the scents of your meat. Then, tie it all up in a big sack and hang that sack out on the end of a large branch. You want the sack to be high enough off the ground that animals cannot reach up to it, and low enough off the branch that animals cannot reach down to it. You also want the area to be clear enough that you can easily keep an eye on everything around you when you are accessing your meat, so you are unlikely to be interrupted and harmed.

Use a large rope to store your meat by tying it to the sack, throwing it over a large branch, and tugging on the rope to pull the sack up toward the branch. Then, secure the end of the rope around the trunk of the tree itself with a knot or a toggle to keep it safely in place until you release it and drop the bag down again for you to access your food with.

CHAPTER 8

Hygiene And Medicine

Hygiene is always important, but it becomes even more important when you are living in the bush. Without proper hygiene, you run the risk of catching an illness and finding yourself in a dangerous or even fatal situation, rapidly. Knowing how to practice proper bush medicine is important, as it ensures that should anything go wrong, you will be able to treat it the best you possibly can. Fortunately, although you may not have access to immediate medical services, there are many things you can do in the bush to help take care of yourself and keep yourself as healthy as possible. In this chapter, we will cover basic bush hygiene and medicine, as well as what to do in the event of common minor injuries.

Personal Hygiene In the Bush

Having a proper hygiene kit for the bush is important. Your hygiene kit should include a toothbrush and toothpaste, a hairbrush, nail clippers, a file, small scissors, a bar of unscented soap, and a razor if you are a male as it will allow you to shave your face if needed. Small cloths that can be used for wiping yourself down and a hand towel are great to have, too.

Every day you should focus on brushing your teeth, brushing your hair, and keeping up with your usual washing routine. However, you should refrain from using soap to wash on a regular basis as doing so can change your scent and make you easier for animals to track. This can make predators curious, and prey fearful, putting you in a bad position in the bush.

Feet are the most important part of hygiene, especially in the bush. When you are bushcrafting, they are put through a lot, from sitting in boots all the time to being rubbed around and exposed to rough terrain as you engage in all the tasks you need to in order to stay healthy and safe. Feet can get small abrasions, bruises, cuts, and blisters. Any of these can quickly fester into serious injuries if you are not careful, so you must always keep your feet as clean as you possibly can. You must also keep your feet dry as wet feet can rapidly develop fungi, which can turn into sores and, as you can probably guess, serious injuries.

If you find yourself unable to access any hygienic products before you leave for the bush, or if you run out, there are a few things you can use in the bush to help you. The smoke from campfires is actually incredibly useful and can be used to wash. Standing in the smoke and letting it get exposed to all parts of you helps neutralize any bacteria that may be lingering anywhere on you and sanitizes your skin and any clothes you may expose to the smoke, too.

You can also use the charcoal from the fire pit to wash your hands and brush your teeth. Or, you can find the bark of a dogwood or a sassafras tree, both of which are quite fibrous and are high in tannic acid. The heightened tannins mean that these two trees are great for cleaning your teeth as they will eliminate any bacteria. Plus, the fibrous nature of them means they can actually scrub your teeth and eliminate any build-up from your mouth.

If using charcoal to wash your hands is not an option or not ideal for you in this moment, you can also use a plant that is high in saponins, which are anti-bacterial and commonly found in everyday soap products. Saponins are readily found in plants like yucca, which are fibrous and excellent for scrubbing hands with.

Which Trees and Plants Are Useful

In the bush, there are many plants you will come across that can help you in different ways. Pines, willow and poplars, black walnut, sassafras, and oaks are all the most likely to give you the best results and are found abundantly nearly everywhere you go. You should also look up a local herbalism guide which will indicate which local flora is useful in medical situations, or in different situations you may encounter in the book. This way, you are educated on plant life in your area, and you can use it as needed.

In the bush, pine trees are great for firewood and building. However, they are also great for medical situations. The sap from pine trees is astringent, antiseptic, anti-inflammatory, and antibacterial. Applying it to wounds helps clean them out and behaves like super glue to hold your wound together. It can also be used to stop bleeding, treat rashes, and to treat sore throats.

The bark of willow trees contains salicin, which turns into salicylic acid in the body. Salicylic acid is great for treating minor aches and pains, arthritis, headaches, and muscle soreness because it acts as an anti-inflammatory. It is especially helpful if you are not particularly used to the demands of bushcraft and find yourself aching at the end of the day, or the next morning.

Poplars are available year-round, making them an excellent tree to rely on. They are easy to spot and can help with an array of things. A poultice made from the leaves of poplar can be used for inflammation and sores; the inner bark can be made into a tea for fevers or upset stomachs; the inner bark can also be chewed if you have a toothache, and it can be used to treat coughs and worms. The easiest way to use poplar is as a tea or a tonic.

Black walnut is great for its ability to kill germs, making it excellent for astringent and antiseptic purposes. Turn it into a poultice to treat a poison ivy rash, or steep it in water to turn it into a wash that will kill bacteria.

Sassafras expels digestive gas, making it an excellent tree to turn into a tea if you are dealing with digestive disorders. The bark itself is also loaded with vitamin C, making it excellent for a natural immune boost in the bush. It can also be turned into a poultice for wounds or rashes. Be careful not to ingest too much sassafras, however, as it can be poisonous in high quantities.

Oaks are the best for building, but they are also great for medicinal situations. White oak in particular, has been used for thousands of years as a medicine. The inner bark is taken from the tree, ground, and decocted to treat any ailment above the neck, ranging from a stuffed nose to a sore throat or a headache. It can also help you prevent excess fluid leakage from the body, meaning it is excellent for runny noses, or if you are dealing with diarrhea. As well, the inner bark of an oak tree can be boiled into a tea and used to clean off wounds before treating them.

Always use the healthiest looking trees available, as they will have the best to offer when it comes to medicinal value. Turn any medicine into a decoction or infusion and consume 8 ounces 3 to 4 times per day, as needed.

Treating Wounds In the Bush

In the bush, treating a wound is vital. Shallow wounds should be first cleaned with an astringent like black walnut or oak; then it should be coated with either honey if you were able to bring any, or fresh pine resin. Get the resin out of the center of the tree, rather than the sap that has been expelled from the tree, as this will be the cleanest kind. Slightly heat it over a fire to make it gooey enough to cover a wound with.

If you have a deep wound, you may need to sew it shut. In this case, you will first clean it, then sew it with a needle that has been sterilized in the fire, and then dress it with pine resin. You will want to cover it with a clean cloth and change the dressing every four to six hours to prevent an infection from developing in the wound.

Dealing With Broken Digits or Limbs

Broken digits or limbs in the bush can be terribly painful and challenging to deal with. Digits are much less of a hassle to deal with as they are not quite as large, and, generally, there is not much you can do for them. If your digit is bent in the wrong direction, you will first need to set it, which means you will need to bend it back in the right direction. As soon as you have, it should find its way back into place. After you have done this, you will want to take a straight, sturdy little branch that is the length of your finger if one of the last two joints was broken, or the length of your hand from your wrist to the tip of your finger if the base joint was broken. Then, you will use a strip of fabric to bind your broken finger to the branch, keeping the branch *over* your hand, not under the palm, to avoid cutting yourself with the end of it whenever you bend your wrist. Keep it this way until the finger is healed.

With arms or legs, you are going to want to evacuate from the bush and seek medical treatment as quickly as possible as these larger bones can rapidly pose a serious threat to anyone who has them. The best way to deal with the broken bone in the field is to cover it with a folded blanket or other soft padded item and carefully tie that item around the broken limb. Then, you will carefully make your way back to civilization, where you can seek support in dealing with that broken limb. Never try to heal a broken limb on your own as they can easily become infected, and if they are set wrong, they can remain damaged for life with no chance of properly healing. In some cases, the limb may no longer be useful or may have to be amputated if it is not set and healed properly.

Healing Gastrointestinal Illness In the Bush

Gastrointestinal illness may mean a day in bed when you are at home, but in the bush, it can rapidly become dangerous. Vomiting and diarrhea can expel much-needed hydration from your body, causing you to rapidly become dehydrated and at risk of fatal illness. This is why people died of grippe before standard medicine protocol was invented. Sassafras infusions should be drank 3-4 times a day in 8-ounce increments, and the ill individual should do their best to continue sipping water throughout the entire day. White oak infusions can also be drunk for diarrhea to hopefully help calm things down and prevent further illness. They should also try to get bites of dried protein whenever possible, as this will ensure that they are able to keep themselves hydrated and nourished. Always thoroughly clean the camp after anyone has been ill to avoid having illness lingering. As well, you will want to be particularly cautious as animals tend to be more aware of other ill mammals based on scent and can become more of a danger when someone is ill.

CHAPTER 9

Leveraging The Environment

Knowing how to use the environment to your benefit is one of the best ways to secure your survival in the bush. The environment can be used in a myriad of ways to support you with survival, whether it be offering food for you to consume or a safe place for you to find shelter. The best way to learn how to leverage the environment is to educate yourself on your local environment and get to know what it is like around you. Pay close attention to what the geography and landscaping are usually like, to what types of plants and animals exist in the area, and to what type of phenomena happen in your area. Knowing how to leverage the environment will go a long way in helping you survive because it ultimately makes survival easier. When you know what to look for, you are able to let the land do much of the work for your survival while you simply have to fill in the gaps.

Educating Yourself On Local Plant Life

The first and biggest thing you can do for yourself is to educate yourself on local plant life. Every area has its own form of vegetation that contributes to the ecosystem, and that can be used in different ways. Educating yourself on the flora local to your environment ensures that you are able to get accurate information on plants that will be relevant for you.

The best way to start educating yourself on local plant life is to invest in a plant guide that is relevant to your local area. Begin reading through it and recognizing which plants are most popular in your area, then highlight them. You do not need to know every single flora in your area, nor do you need to know how all of it works. However, you do need to know the ones that are going to be most likely to help you. Look for flora that can be safely consumed, as well as flora that can be used for medical purposes for treating injuries and for treating illnesses. You should have a few different plants identified for each circumstance. Next, get out in the field and practice identifying those plants so that you can see them for yourself and get comfortable with identifying them and locating them in the wild. This way, if you are ever caught in a survival situation, it is easy for you to locate what you need.

If you want to feel even more confident in your local flora, you can always work with a herbalist. Local herbalists are educated in local flora and vegetation, and therefore they have an abundance of information and answers on local plant life. Many will offer plant walks in nearby forests and parks and, on those walks, will help you confidently identify important plants. They can also educate you on how to safely and sustainably harvest those plants and use them if need be, and you can ask as many questions as you need or want.

Properly and Safely Identifying Plants

It is important that you learn to properly and safely identify any plants you are considering using, as many plants are known for having plants that look similar but are highly poisonous. For example, grapes are safe to consume, but pokeweed berries that look like greats are toxic and become even more toxic as they mature, to the point where consumption can be fatal. Never eat just anything you see, and always be absolutely confident that what you are eating is safe to eat.

The best way to properly and safely identify plants is to practice doing so, especially with the guide of someone with greater skill who can confirm one way or another if you have properly identified said plant. Going out in the field with someone who knows what they are talking about means that they can help you recognize certain signs or indications that allow you to tell a safe plant apart from a dangerous one. You should do this several times over and keep notes in your local plant life book if need be to ensure that you are prepared to safely and confidently identify the local flora in a survivalist situation if need be.

Another way to protect yourself is to educate yourself on the poisonous plants in your area, and any poisonous plants that tend to look like the ones you intend to rely on if you find yourself in a survivalist situation. As they say, "keep your friends close, but your enemies closer." The better you are at identifying dangerous plants, the less likely you will be to accidentally engage with them and find yourself ill or even dead as a result.

Consuming and Storing Edible Plants

Most plants that are edible can be consumed as is, though some may taste better when cooked. In a survivalist setting, you can harvest plant matter directly from a plant itself, though it is important to do so in a sustainable way. Harvesting plant matter in a sustainable way ensures that you are able to continue harvesting from the same plant over and over and that you do not slowly deplete any given area of a certain type of plant. Typically, plants should be harvested above the root and near any "joints" that you may see in the leaves or stems.

All harvested plants should be washed in fresh, filtered water, as you never know what has been on or around that plant. Animal urine can contaminate plants and transfer bacteria and parasites onto them, rendering them dangerous for you to eat. If you are picking from a bush, always pick high up where the plant is likely to remain less bothered by animals. Practice care when harvesting to avoid being bitten or stung by an insect that could be harmful in and of itself.

If you are not going to consume something right away, store it in a clean, dry, cool space for up to a couple of days. Berries, for example, could be stored inside of a loosely sealed container in the shade or in a shallow, cool stream. Green plant matter can either be dried and used to season meats or other foods with or can be stored in the same manner as berries would be until you are ready to consume them.

Using the Landscape to Build a Camp

Aside from using local vegetation for medicine and food, there are other ways to use the landscape to your advantage. One great way is to use the landscape itself to help you build a camp. While you do need to watch for the 5 W's, it is helpful to use the landscape to help you in as many ways as possible. Avoid setting up camp "just anywhere" and set camp up somewhere that is already relatively cleared out, or that has something you can use for setting up camp. Look for trees that are the right height, branches that are going to allow you to easily hang things, and water that is easy to access and clean.

When it comes to your survival, the last thing you want to have to worry about is trying to clear out a proper campsite so that you can access everything you need. Having to cut away trees, clear out brush, or clean off the dirt itself so that you can use the landscape properly requires work, and work uses up calories, and calories are harder to come by in the bush. You need to preserve as much of your energy and time as you possibly can so that you are able to use it on other, more important things such as finding water and food and keeping yourself warm, hydrated, and fed.

Another thing you should consider when you are getting ready to set up camp is how easy it will be to set your food preservation site and cook site up. A well-placed camp should be able to be a part of a triangle, with your cook site and your food preservation site all kept 100 yards apart. If you are going to have to climb any nasty hills or do any excessive or treacherous walking to get to these areas, you are going to find yourself at greater risk. You want to try to find an area that is going to be easy to live in and navigate so that you can make it as effortless as possible for you to survive. As it is, survival is going to take more energy and effort than you can possibly imagine. The easier you can make it for yourself, the better.

Getting Creative With the Landscape

Speaking of making things easier through the landscape, it can be helpful to look for other ways to make use of the landscape, too. More often than not, the earth is formed in such a way that it can effortlessly help us achieve anything we desire, whether that be to create shelter, hunt or prepare food, or gather water for drinking, cleaning, and cooking.

Before you embark on any survival venture, stop and survey the landscape. What do you see? What might be able to help you make your job easier? How might you be able to achieve more with less? Consider looking for trees that are already perfectly shaped to help you set up your tarp or tent, or for branches that are already the perfect height for you to prepare your game. Look for parts of the water that are easy to access or runways that are already made so that you can easily move around the forest you are currently residing in.

When we spend our entire lives in urban environments, it can be easy to forget that nature itself has its own system going on inside of it. When you step into that system, there is no need to reinvent it or try to manipulate it to be your way. Doing so will only use up your energy and make it more challenging for you to survive. Focus instead on meshing into the system that already exists and using it to your advantage. Get creative. Look for ways to make things work, and don't be afraid to make adaptations as needed. One of the greatest survival skills anyone can have is the ability to adapt their plans as needed and shift into a system that works for their present situation. When you know how to get creative and make things work for what you need, you increase your chances of survival tenfold.

CONCLUSION

Surviving in the bush will not be the easiest task you will ever come up against, should you find yourself in this situation. There are many challenges you will face, many hardships you will have to overcome, and many adaptations you will need to make. If you do find yourself in a survival situation, one thing I want to warn you against is what will likely be the greatest challenge you will face. That is, your mind.

Your mind is a wildly powerful tool, and when it is fixed to help you survive, it will do wonders. However, your mind can and will go through phases where it seems virtually impossible for you to survive at all. You are going to wonder if it is worth it, what you are doing this for, and if it is even possible for you to survive in the long run. You may become anxious from all of the changes and stress, depressed from all of the loss, or angry from everything you are being faced with. This is all normal and natural. You must learn to ride the natural waves of your emotions while still charging forward if you are going to survive, and you must learn how to always put your survival above anything else.

This book is an excellent resource to help you learn how to survive in the bush, but the truth of the matter is that your memory is not going to function the same under the stress of a survivalist situation. You would be best to keep a printed copy of this safely tucked into your grab and go bag so that if you do find yourself in the bush, you also have access to all of the information right here in these pages. One small mistake in the bush can be dangerous and even fatal, so having this available to keep you on top of things is important.

I also encourage you to keep going from here. Do not make this the only way you educate yourself for survival. Keep researching, reading, and looking to understand everything you can. You can start by checking out my other titles, *Survival 101: Beginner's Guide 2021*, *Survival 101: Food Storage,* and *Survival 101: Raised Bed Gardening.* There are many guides out there, all of which will give you valuable information to help you discover exactly what you need to know in order to survive. Be sure to research your locale, as well, to discover what your terrain is like, where the best areas for setting up camp are, and how to survive once you get there. The more you can educate yourself on local threats and risks, the easier it will be for you to prepare yourself and protect yourself if you ever find yourself in a situation where you need to.

Before you go, I ask that you please take a moment to review *Survival 101: Bushcraft* on Amazon Kindle. Your honest feedback would be greatly appreciated, as it will help others like you discover how they, too, can survive in the bush. It will also help me write more great titles for you.

Thank you, and good luck! Stay safe out there.

Survival 101: Beginner's Guide

2021

The Complete Guide To Urban And Wilderness Survival

Rory Anderson

INTRODUCTION

None of us could have possibly anticipated the disaster that has come with 2020, nor the state it would leave us in. Between the growing threat of the pandemic and the crashing economy, there is plenty of reason to have doubts about our modern system. Right now is the perfect time to begin developing your survival skills. That way, you'll know exactly how to protect yourself should things get any worse than they already are.

Perhaps the most significant threat we are all facing right now is the growing economic crisis, as well as the pressure it is putting on our current way of life. From a lack of income to messed up supply chains, it is increasingly more challenging to access anything you need for survival these days. While it may not be a big deal that you cannot directly go out and buy new clothes, furniture, and frivolous supplies, it is a growing concern that the strain is reaching deep into our food supplies, our hygienic supplies, and even our access to medications and other health and first aid requirements.

As of right now, there is no clear end in sight, nor is there any plausible solution that seems to be capable of repairing the damage. While many who are in charge continue to spout off about possible ideas and attempt to affirm that everything is fine, it is clear that everything is *not* fine. We don't know how much worse it might get. In an ideal world, we may be able to trust our government to protect us. Still, based on current conditions and experiences, many people are growing rightfully doubtful and distrustful in their government. So, if you cannot trust society, the current state of affairs, supply chains, or your government, what is left for you to do? *Survive.*

We are like any other species when faced with a threat to our very survival. Including the breakdown of our current system, it will all come down to an "every man for himself" situation. This may seem extravagant, but the reality is that hundreds of thousands of people are faced with this every single year. From wildfires, hurricanes, and other natural disasters, to pandemics, economic crashes, and the implementation of police states in some areas, humans have been granted rude awakening after rude awakening. That is that while the current system and connection of supply chains may provide you with convenience and comfort when they are all eliminated, you are left with *nothing*. If you don't know how to survive without them, the minute an emergency arises, you will find yourself staring down a serious threat and having no idea what to do about it. Only those who educate themselves will survive the deadliest of emergencies. If you want to be one of them, you have to take your education seriously.

Survival 101: Beginner's Guide 2020 will help you navigate our current state of affairs. It is also designed to help you navigate *any* state of crisis. Whether the emergency is mild, moderate, or extreme, you will discover everything you need to know. Please note that while this book will support hobbyists who want to prepare for the future, this book is certainly not geared toward hobbyists. This book is designed to help in real-life emergency survival situations. Everything you will discover in this book will tell you precisely what you need to do to survive any crisis you happen across.

While much of this book is written specifically for the purpose of surviving in a natural environment, I realize that you might currently be residing in an urban setting. For that reason, there will be information on urban survival and escaping urban situations as needed, should you find yourself in that situation. Please be sure to educate yourself based on your current circumstances so that you can secure your safety and your future.

Before you dive in, I want to take a moment to thank you for choosing *Survival 101: Beginner's Guide*. This book is one of many on the market today, and I am grateful and humbled that you have chosen mine. Thank you. Please, enjoy it.

CHAPTER 1
Preparing To Survive

Our present society continues to revolve around broken systems and overdrawn supply chains. While these systems work perfectly when everything is going "as it should," the minute something goes wrong, they rapidly break down. With that being said, the systems have worked, and they have managed to provide us with many excellent tools that we can use to our advantage. Using what is available to you is the first key to surviving. If you live in an urban environment, you have a lot available to you. While it may be challenging for you to access it during the pandemic, much of it is still accessible. It will provide you with a means of safety and survival should anything else go wrong.

Preparing yourself to survive requires you to first educate yourself on what survival will look like for your unique situation. Developing this knowledge will help you recognize the risks and considerations unique to your situation. It will help you maintain a clear action plan for any emergency level you need to address. Remember that survival does not come with a one-size-fits-all solution, so you need to plan for *your* unique circumstances. I will tell you how.

Gauging Your Current Situation

The first order of business when it comes to survival is gauging your current situation so that you know exactly what it is that you need to do to survive. Become aware of what your current lifestyle looks like, where you gather all your supplies, where you store your supplies, and what your exit routes are. What possible risk-factors you face based on your unique circumstances. This way, you know what to be aware of, consider, and manage when addressing emergencies.

If you live in a rural environment, your risk factor could be that you lose contact with the rest of the world so you cannot easily access food, supplies, medical assistance, or any external assistance, should anything go wrong. Alternatively, if you live in an urban environment, your risk factor could be that you do not have enough space to store large amounts of survival tools, your local supply chains for food and supplies could run dry, and your environment could collapse. You could end up hurt, or grid-locked and unable to leave in a timely fashion. Often, the most significant risk to those in rural settings is the risk of being cut off from the rest of the world, which creates a significant threat. At the same time, those in urban environments run the risk of getting too comfortable and not knowing how to protect themselves in case of an emergency. In either scenario, your livelihood could be at serious risk.

As you assess your current situation, pay close attention to how you are accessing the five requirements for survival. Water, shelter, fire, food, and safety need to be your priorities in a survival situation. Fire is considered mandatory for survival as it helps maintain your core temperature. Fire also provides you with a reliable cooking source and a tool that can help people locate you if you find yourself lost and waiting on search and rescue teams.

Once you have defined your current situation, you are going to look for all possible risk factors and then create a plan for how to minimize those risk factors. You need to have a plan for how you are going to secure your five requirements for survival. Having a clear, well-crafted plan ensures that no matter what happens, you feel confident that you can advocate for and take care of your survival. This way, you are never left relying on anyone else and possibly growing ill, injured, or dying as a result.

Measuring Emergency Levels

Measuring emergency levels is vital as it allows you to determine how you execute your response plan. For mild emergencies, the execution of your response will be far less intense than it will be in extreme emergencies. You need to know how to measure and monitor emergencies confidently so that you can take the response that feels right *for you*. Realize that everyone will speculate what they believe the intended threat level is, and that you will likely hear about these speculations all over mass media and throughout society. You need to personally decide what you believe the risk factor is, based on your best-educated guess, and respond accordingly.

Waiting for the authorities to provide you with adequate information regarding your risk level has left many people in dire situations that directly threatened their livelihood. For example, in 2020, it was speculated that if every country had taken the pandemic seriously just two weeks sooner, we would have seen less than half of the impact we see right now. Unfortunately, government and authorities do not always respond to things promptly, so relying on them is not always the right solution. You need to become confident in relying on yourself and your own best judgment to protect yourself in case of an emergency since you alone are responsible for your survival.

In terms of emergencies, there are three levels of emergencies to look out for:

- mild emergencies, which are sometimes called level three emergencies
- moderate emergencies, which are sometimes called level two emergencies
- extreme emergencies, which are sometimes called level one emergencies.

Mild emergencies, also called level three emergencies, are considered isolated, contained critical incidents. These might include something like a single non-life-threatening injury, a fire that was contained or extinguished, or something else that would be considered an emergency, but that is controlled and not actively spreading. At home, this might include a fall, a broken bone, or a flood. In your town, this might include a nearby flood, a single building such as a grocery store or a school catching fire, or something similar. Based on our current emergency with COVID-19, level three of this emergency would have been when the illness was first located in other countries but had not yet spread, and was not yet escalated to a crisis or a pandemic.

Moderate or level two emergencies are considered situational crises. Situational crises are ones that are not developing or worsening. Still, they do require more significant assistance to protect yourself in these circumstances. For example, if a large portion of your home was on fire or there was an uncontained fire in your house, if you had fallen and seriously hurt yourself and were unable to get up to retrieve help, or if you were ill with something like bacterial meningitis. More significant floods and nearby wildfires can also be considered level two emergencies.

A level one emergency or a crisis is a state in which something significant is going on. Hurricanes, major floods, tsunamis, uncontrollable wildfires, and other natural disasters that pose a major threat to peoples' wellbeing are recognized as level one emergencies. Man-made disasters such as active war zones, police states, and pandemics also classify as a level one emergency. In all of these scenarios, you are immediately cut off from all five things you need for survival and are required to manage your own survival until society can come back together *if* society is able to come back together.

Emergencies You Are Most Likely to Come Across

The exact types of emergencies you should be aware of and prepared for depending on where you come from and what your climate and geographical regions are. Each area will have unique natural threats that can rapidly evolve into emergencies and threaten your survival.

If you live in a cold climate or near the arctic circle, you are likely to face emergencies such as wind storms, freezing water, and exposure. Wind storms can be incredibly cold, can blow snow around and create white-outs or blizzards, and can damage things such as trees and create hazards from falling objects. Freezing water can make it impossible for you to source drinking water, or could cause illness or death if you were to fall in and experience hypothermia or frostbite. In some cases, this can happen in mere minutes. Exposure is a danger that can lead to hypothermia and frostbite. Avalanches are another possibility in cold climates, particularly if you live near the mountains. As well, you should consider the fact that food and water supplies may be cut off if you cannot get any imported to you and could be hard to locate due to hunting and foraging becoming far more challenging in the winter.

If you live in the desert, monsoon, drought, haboob, and microbursts can be considered threats to your survival. A monsoon is a heavy rainstorm that typically occurs later in the day and can lead to rapid flooding. This is due to the amount of rain that falls and the fact that the ground is too dry to absorb all of the water adequately. Drought occurs when there is limited or no rainfall for long periods and can lead to dehydration. It can also make growing crops much more challenging. During periods of drought, it can also be hot and dry, which can lead to heatstroke or even death from overheating. Haboobs are giant walls of dust and dirt that can grow as tall as 3,000 feet and stretch miles long, and dust storms often accompany them. The storm itself can put you at risk from exposure by destroying air quality, and they can also damage crops, homes, and other environmental features. Microbursts, on the other hand, are incredibly strong concentrated winds that can tear things down in their path. Microbursts are similar to tornados, but they do not spin in circles as tornados do.

The tropics are well-known for having hurricanes or tropical storms, earthquakes, floods, and windstorms. They can also get monsoon weather, which can increase the risk of flooding and flood-related damages. These natural disasters can be dangerous and routinely cause injuries and fatalities every single year.

Heavily forested areas like what is seen on the west coast of North America and the grassy regions like the prairies or the Midwest are often at the highest risk of dealing with wildfires and earthquakes. Regions that have mountains are at risk of landslides and, during winter seasons, avalanches. Flooding is also frequent in wet forested areas such as those seen along the west coast of North America.

If you live immediately along the coastline, you are at considerable risk of water-related threats. Tsunamis can be a threat, as can hurricanes or earthquakes that lead to flooding. On individual islands, such as those in Hawaii, there is also the risk of a volcano erupting and rendering entire areas of land unlivable for extended periods.

Knowing what types of natural disasters are likely to strike your region allows you to properly prepare for the threats you may face. You should make a plan for how you will face each and every possible disaster in your area, both natural and man-made, so that you have a plan for any unique circumstance you may come up against. Backup plans are also ideal, as they can kick into effect and keep everyone on the same page in case your original plan does not pan out. You find yourself in need of something more significant to protect you.

Preparing for Extreme Emergencies

You and your family need to prepare for extreme emergencies. Being prepared for an extreme emergency ensures that you are ready for mild and moderate emergencies, too, should one occur. Preparing for an emergency requires you to consider four things: your resources, your plan of operations, your escape, and your long term survival. If you can adequately prepare for all four of these aspects of your livelihood, you will have a much stronger chance of surviving any emergency you happen across.

Planning for emergencies requires you to know exactly what resources you need, and how many of those resources you need so that you can accommodate for every person in your household. You need enough food, water, shelter, clothes, medicine, hygiene products, and protection for every single person in your family, as well as anything else you can reasonably bring to aid and simplify survival measures. In long term survival situations, there is no way you will be able to tote in large amounts of food or water for your survival, so you will want to have a plan for how you are going to acquire and sterilize food and water, too. For example, you will want to have hunting supplies and water purifier on hand so that you can safely harvest and consume food and water in a natural environment.

Your plan of operations should be a detailed plan for how you are going to survive in any situation you find yourself in. This includes how you are going to escape if you need to, where you are going to go, and what you are going to do when you get there. Your order of operations is essential as it keeps you organized and focused on doing the most essential things required for your survival in the most important order. You must secure the most critical things first, as everything else can come next. For example, you need to acquire water before food because the average human can survive three weeks without food but only three days without water. Before anything else, though, you need to secure shelter because if your core body temperature drops, you will not be able to secure anything else. Doing everything in proper rule, then, is critical.

In addition to knowing how you are going to survive an emergency, you need to know how you are going to escape one. Many situations will require you to escape to a safer environment until your present environment is safer to return to. Knowing how you will escape is critical, as your survival skills are virtually useless if you are trapped in a dangerous situation. In a rural or coastal setting, your escape might include where you will go and how you will get away should a tornado, hurricane, or another significant storm roll in. In an urban environment, your plan of getaway might consist of how you will get away if you need to leave the urban environment, and everything is at risk of becoming grid-locked. You will also need to consider *when* you will time your escape, as you want to make sure that you go before it is too late. Of course, you do not want to leave too early and find yourself having to rely on survival skills long before you need to, because this can lead to a depletion of your resources.

Finally, you need to prepare for long term survival. If returning to your home is not an option for extended periods of time, you need to feel confident that you can survive until then. Having a plan for how you will support your survival for an extended period ensures that you can survive for as long as you need and that you do not perish in the woods due to a lack of survival knowledge and skills.

The Skills You Will Need

Bushcraft and wilderness skills are vital for your ability to survive an emergency. Knowing how to make a fire, navigate the wilderness, trap, track, build shelter, and use wilderness tools will help you accomplish everything you need to survive. I discuss all of these skills in far greater detail in my book *Survival 101: Bushcraft*. Gardening is another great skill to have, as well as knowing how to preserve food for extended periods of time. I discuss these topics in my books *Survival 101: Raised Bed Gardening 2021* and *Survival 101: Food Storage*. Foraging and scavenging for food in a natural environment is also a great skill to have as it ensures that you are able to select a variety of food sources and that you do not have to rely solely on animal proteins or wait excessive periods of time for your food to start growing.

The key to surviving in the wilderness and living off the land is realizing that there will be multiple skills that are relevant to your survival. Not only are you going to need to know about *what* has to be done, but you are also going to need to know-*how*. This means that by learning how to build a shelter, for example, you also need to know how to use an ax and a saw properly, how to properly secure things in place, and how to use other resources such as rope and knot tying to create a safe environment. The more skills you know, the more likely you will be to survive in the wilderness for as long as you need to. We will discuss all of these skills, and more, between *Chapter 3: The First Five,* and *Chapter 5: The 34 Tasks of Survival*.

CHAPTER 2

Key Terms

As you read through the remainder of this book, you are going to come across many terms that may seem unusual or foreign to you. These terms are commonly used in survival situations to define certain circumstances, tasks, or objects that are relevant to a survival scenario. Before we dig any deeper into survival itself, we are going to discuss what these key terms are and why they are pertinent to your survival.

Area of Operation (AO)

Area of Operation (AO) defines the area where your operations take place. This term was first described by the U.S. armed forces parlance to establish an operational area where the armed forces would be conducting their operational tasks. In an emergency, your AO refers to the area you are leaving, the area you are going to, and the area you will be passing through to get there. Your AO will define the entire area in which you will be surviving. This includes where you will sleep, cook, fetch water, hunt, and otherwise live for the duration of the emergency.

You should have a clearly defined AO, and no one should leave the AO at any given time without a clear procedure and reason as to why they are leaving. Leaving without a proper plan could result in someone getting lost or becoming exposed to unexpected threats due to being in an area that you are not used to or comfortable in. There should also be a clearly defined set of trails and roads within the AO that will determine where you go at all times, and everyone should stay on those trails and paths. Leaving them could result in becoming lost or injured as well.

A-Team

Your A-Team, when it comes to survival, relates to every single person who will be coming with you in a survival setting, and it refers to the hierarchy or operational order inside of that team. While you might think the only people you will care about in a survivalist setting will be those in your immediate household, it is ideal to have at least one or two other families who will be joining you. You should all have a clear plan for how you will survive once you reach the wilderness, and what each of you is going to do to aid survival. There is strength in numbers, even in the wilderness, so having additional members of your A-Team should always be welcomed and supported.

Having a clearly defined hierarchy in your A-Team ensures that everyone knows who to listen to and what their role is for the survival of the team. The last thing you need is to come up against dominance struggles or miscommunications in the wilderness, so you want to have this sorted out beforehand. Everyone should do what they know best, which means the leaders of your group should include people who are knowledgeable about survival and who are capable of giving orders and guiding the team in a practical but compassionate manner. Aside from that, you should have people committed to cooking, hunting, foraging, fetching water, gardening, building, and performing other survival-related tasks. While one person can certainly take on multiple tasks, it is essential to avoid giving one person more functions than anyone else. This can lead to that person burning out and everyone suffering as a result. Everyone should take on an equal task load and do their part to contribute to the survival of everyone at the camp.

Bug Out Hideout Site (BOHS)

A Bug Out Hideout Site (BOHS) is essential for you to survive an emergency. The military first described the BOHS in the 1950s. Now, it is used by the preparedness community as a way to define the location that a family will escape to should anything go wrong.

Ideally, your BOHS should be identified in advance and should be well-known by those who will be surviving with you, and *only* by those who will be surviving with you. If possible, a well-developed BOHS will already have shelter in place, and everyone who will be surviving there should know how to get there safely and navigate the area around it.

You should define your BOHS in advance and get comfortable in the area, as this will increase your confidence in surviving in this space. When everyone is clear and familiar with the area, it is easier to execute survival tasks because everyone is already familiar with where everything is. Therefore, it is quicker to get yourselves set up and cover your essentials faster. The looming pressure of an emergency can make traveling and surviving more challenging, so having this confidence in your BOHS location means you do not have to rely on your logic during an emergency because it all comes back through memory.

Emergency Rallying Point (ERP)

An emergency rallying point (ERP) is where you are going to rally in the case of an emergency. You will define your ERP based on what emergencies you are likely to face in your environment and where the safest rallying point would be. You should have an ERP for your household, and an ERP for anyone who would be going to your BOHS with you, including any members of your A-Team. This way, the members of your household can gather quickly in mild to moderate emergencies. The members of your family and other A-Team members can gather quickly in moderate to extreme emergencies where evacuation is required. Your ERP will be far closer than your BOHS, and you and your A-Team will travel from the ERP to the BOHS together to ensure safety and security.

Grab and Go Bag (GnG Bag)

A Grab and Go Bag (GnG Bag) is essential for an emergency where you do not have enough time to pack up all of your gear and head to your ERP or your BOHS. In some emergencies, such as natural disasters, there is no time for you to gather everything and head to your ERP, so you must grab your GnG Bag and go.

Your GnG Bag should have the absolute essentials for your survival, including things like:

- Ready to eat non-perishable food
- Drinking water
- Solar-powered phone charger
- Crank radio
- Crank flashlight
- Extra batteries
- Personal toiletries
- Personal medications
- First-aid kit
- Copy of the emergency plan
- Documents including insurance papers and personal identification
- Garbage bags
- Moist towelettes

- Cash in small bills
- Seasonal clothing
- Emergency blanket
- Sturdy footwear
- Dust mask
- Whistle
- Flare.

You should also have a "help/OK" sign to display in your window so that if you are trapped in your home during an emergency situation, you can display this in your window for safety. This way, if emergency crews come by and see "help," they know that you or someone inside of your dwelling is in need of immediate help, and they can prioritize helping you.

Immediate Rallying Point (IRP)

An immediate rallying point (IRP) differs from the ERP because it will be closer to home. An ERP should be removed enough from your immediate vicinity that if an emergency strikes, you can remove yourself from that emergency space before it harms you. For example, if you have a few hours or days of warning before a wildfire comes through your town, you can use your ERP. In some scenarios, the crisis may not be large enough to warrant leaving your immediate vicinity, or it may be so large that it is now too dangerous to leave. For these scenarios, you need an IRP which will be in your immediate vicinity. An underground storm shelter beneath your house would be a great example of an IRP.

You should have two IRP's defined: one for scenarios where you can stay in your own home and one for situations where you must leave it. Have a clearly defined IRP so that everyone in your home knows where to find everyone else. This is especially important if you have a large household, as certain disasters can shred homes and leave various rooms a threat. You would not want to lose someone in a different room of your house because you did not know they were there. If you cannot stay in your home, your locale will have storm shelters or emergency shelters where you can go for safekeeping. Determine which shelter you and your family will use in case of an emergency so that if any of you are not home when the emergency strikes, you can feel confident that you will all find your way back together. Hopefully, you will be able to leave the IRP for the ERP and the BOHS after things settle down.

CHAPTER 3
The First Five

As soon as you find yourself in a survival situation, you must immediately focus on fulfilling the five things that are most important to your survival. These five things include water, shelter, fire, food, and safety. Without either of these five things, you face the risk of becoming severely ill or even dying as they are all crucial to your survival. It is essential to understand that how you access and secure such things in an urban environment will differ from a natural environment. Knowing how to obtain these five things for yourself and your A-Team will ensure that you remain safe and that you can protect yourself under any circumstance.

The First Five Urban VS. Off-Grid Environments

Naturally, how you secure water, shelter, fire, food, and safety is going to differ between urban and natural or off-grid environments. In an urban environment, some of what you need is supplied by the city you live in and will already be standing. In contrast, in a natural environment, you will be solely responsible for accessing everything you need.

In an urban situation, you are going to need to account for the fact that you have limited space. However, you will have access to shelter that is already built and secured, which makes it easier for you to secure a place to stay. You will need to check the quality of your shelter to ensure it is safe, though, and protected from external dangers. If you are not, you will need to make immediate repairs or adjustments to secure your safety and survival.

Aside from the shelter, most urban environments have built-in supply chains for water, food, electricity, and safety. When you come across a survival emergency, all four of these things can disappear, and, in some cases, the shelter can, too. For example, during a hurricane, you might find your accommodation damaged, which means you need to find somewhere else to stay.

When your supply chains for water, food, electricity, and safety are destroyed, you have to discover a new means of securing water, food, fire, and protection. If you are lucky, you may already have a stocked pantry with purified water that you stored in case of an emergency. However, you are still going to need to source as much of these things as you possibly can. In a long term emergency, this may include sending two people out to a nearby rural environment to fish or trap animal proteins and forage for plant proteins. Water can also be challenging to source in an urban environment, particularly if your water lines have been damaged, shut off, or contaminated. Ideally, you should be able to access water from a nearby river or stream. However, you should assume that it is contaminated from urban runoff sources, so you will need to purify it properly. In a situation where your electricity is off, you will need to use fire for cooking and heat. During these types of emergencies, take note of whether or not you have any natural gas supplied to your house. If you do, check to make sure there are no gas leaks, as gas leaks lead to fatalities. As well, make sure there are no active powerlines or livewires, which could lead to a dangerous or fatal electric shock. Finally, you need to consider your safety in an urban environment when it comes to external forces. If you find yourself in a police state, you need to consider your safety against the authorities. If you find yourself in a long term survival situation, you need to be cautious of looters who will rob people of their resources in a means to secure their survival.

If you are not in an urban environment when a survival emergency strikes, or if you have left your urban environment, you are going to have to be single-handedly responsible for everything associated with your survival. You need to build shelter, secure water, build a fire, harvest food, and protect yourself from any threats in the environment. Ultimately, you will be starting from scratch using any tools and resources you were able to bring and all of the resources available to you in the wilderness. Fortunately, since we are mammals, everything you need to survive is underfoot. Hence, even if you have to escape with nothing but the clothes off your back, there is still hope for survival.

Shelter

The shelter is the first thing you need to secure, as daytime rapidly turns into nighttime, and nighttime is when you are at your most significant risk. In any environment, the night is when temperatures drop. If you are already enduring cold weather, these drops can be deadly.

In an urban environment, nighttime is when people are asleep. Therefore, they are least prepared for anything that might happen. If a natural disaster strikes, you will be less alert and prepared, as will everyone around you. In terms of human dangers, the night is when people are more likely to ambush you or attempt to rob you, making it a more significant threat. In a natural environment, nighttime temperatures get even cooler since your heat will not be entirely as secure as an urban shelter would be. Animals who tend to hunt at night will have an advantage on you by having better eyesight, sharper senses, and a more exceptional ability to attack and defend themselves during the evening. Having a safe place to stay is crucial to protect you against any nighttime threats.

If you are surviving in an urban setting, there are four types of shelter you can use. Ideally, you should remain in your home as your primary shelter, which should be your absolute goal. The only time you should leave your home is if it becomes damaged or has to for some dire reason. Otherwise, this is where you should remain. The second possible shelter, if you have to leave your home, would be to stay with a family member or a friend in their home. This way, you know who you are staying with, and feel comfortable supporting each other and surviving together. If a family member or friend is not possible, you may be able to stay with a neighbor who has room for you. However, you should beware of the fact that trying to stay with a neighbor could be hit or miss. The third option would be to stay in a local shelter. When natural disasters strike, municipal governments will set up local shelters for people to remain in if their own homes are uninhabitable, and you can stay there. Note that these environments will offer minimal means for independence, and you will have to abide by the rules, which may or may not contradict what you believe to be right for your survival. The fourth option for shelter would be to find an empty home that no one lives in and take it over as your own for the duration of your survival emergency. However, this should be an absolute last resort as it can lead to legal issues and other dangers, such as the homeowner removing you by force. Finally, if you cannot secure a sanctuary where you are, you should retreat to a natural environment and secure shelter there.

In the wilderness, securing shelter requires some consideration. Namely, you need to pick a spot that factors in the five W's which are necessary for survival in any wilderness situation. The five W's are wood, water, weather, widowmakers, and wildlife.

The best location to build your shelter is one with plenty of wood available. Wood is an excellent building material and fuel for fires. Plus, building your shelter in a forest means the trees will protect you from most weather fronts.

Water is essential for your survival, so you need to set up camp somewhere where you can easily access water, as you do not want to be dragging gallons of water along a lengthy, steep path back to shelter. However, make sure the water is downhill from where you are so you are not at risk of floods or sleeping on continually moist grounds.

You must take the weather seriously, as the weather is the number one cause for people dying in the wilderness. Death by exposure is severe, painful, and happens rapidly. Consider the climate of the area you are in and plan your shelter accordingly. You need to be safely shaded away from the hot sun, protected from rainfall, and kept warm and insulated in a cold or snowy environment. Build accordingly and build quickly. The most accessible shelter to build for wet weather is a lean-to, though A-frame tents work well. To construct a lean-to, you will simply hang a tarp from four trees, with one side of the tarp being higher than the other. If your tarp is long enough, or if you have an extra tarp, you can run the lower end of the tarp to the ground to give you a comfortable, dry spot at the back of the lean-to. Build an A-Frame tent by finding five Y-shaped logs and one straight log. You want to prop your five Y-shaped logs up by having the first, third, and fifth logs with the Y-shape down so that they have one single branch end up in the air. The second and fourth logs should be upside down with two arms in the air and strapped to the first and fifth log. This way, you can stabilize your structure. Lay the single, long log in the crook of the Y-shaped logs, so it runs across the top of the shelter like a roof beam. You can then cover the entire shelter with a tarp if you have one. If not, you can use spruce needle branches with the needles still on, leafy branches, twigs, moss, and long grasses to help build a roof over your shelter. In particularly wet or cold situations, you should combine a tarp with a naturally-built roof to provide insulation and protect you from the damp weather. If you are in a cold condition, digging a small cave into a snowbank is the best option for shelter. Refrain from digging it out to be too deep, as this can cause the snow to collapse and can trap you inside, causing certain death.

Widowmakers are natural threats in the wilderness that can instantly injure or kill you. For example, if you build a snow hut that is too deep and the snow collapses, you have died as the result of a widowmaker. Trees and branches that are starting to fall over can fall at random or with a small wind gust, and they can also injure or kill anyone in their path. Rockslides, mudslides, and avalanches can also be widowmakers, so you will want to assess your risk for these threats and protect yourself if need be. Never set up camp in a spot where any of these threats are looming, as they can lead to accidental injury or death.

Finally, you need to consider wildlife when you are in the wilderness. Avoid building your camp in a space where wildlife frequents. "Wildlife highways" as they are called stomped-out paths and clearings in the wilderness, where a variety of wildlife frequents. Camping too close to one could result in untimely or unwanted meetings between you and wild animals, which could pose a severe threat to your safety. Camping nearby to these wildlife highways is a good idea as it puts you relatively close to a spot where you can easily trap wildlife for food, but do not get too close. It is a good idea to educate yourself on local wildlife, so you know what to expect and how to protect yourself properly. So you know what type of wildlife is available to harvest and eat if you find yourself in a survival emergency.

Water

After you secure shelter, water is the next most crucial thing. The only time water comes before accommodation is if you will be escaping an urban environment to survive, in which case both water and food should come first if you are capable of securing purified water and non-perishable, ready-to-eat food items. Otherwise, locating a source of water becomes your next order of operation.

In an urban environment, you can generally source water directly from the tap, even during emergency situations. Even so, you should keep an ample amount of bottled or canned water on hand so that if you ever find yourself unable to access water, you can safely consume the water you have stored. More often than not, government and rescue organizations will come through with a safe quantity of drinking water within hours or days of an emergency striking. With that being said, they will have limited supply. They may not be able to find you, or you may not be able to find them, so you need to be prepared to source your water if and when your water supply runs out. If you cannot access water from your tap, look for a nearby stream, creek, or river. Lakes, ponds, or man-made waterbodies will work. Still, the water is more likely to be contaminated, so be sure to properly purify it first.

It is essential that no matter where you harvest water from in an urban environment that you assume that water is highly contaminated. Urban environments have a variety of chemical runoffs that contaminate all water sources, including the rain. Tap water is treated for these runoffs, but in an emergency, situation treatment can become faulty or ineffective. For that reason, you need to treat *all* water if you are facing a moderate to extreme emergency. Having testing strips handy at home is essential in an urban environment as it will allow you to check your water for chemicals. You should test tap water to monitor that it continues to be safe to use, and stop using it or start treating it the minute it becomes unsafe. If you are going to need to survive for an extended period of time, and have access to multiple water sources, test each source to see which will be the cleanest. You will still need to purify it, but this will ensure that you are least likely to drink contaminated water and wind up sick.

In a natural environment, water needs to be sourced from a natural water source. Springwater from creeks, streams, rivers, and waterfalls are ideal as the movement of the water prevents bacteria and parasites from building up in them. Water such as lakes, ponds, and large pools are often the least safe, as they can become contaminated, and there is no way for the contaminants to move out. However, if that is all you have access to, then it will have to do.

Always assume that all water in a natural setting is contaminated and treat it to avoid getting sick. Even if you are drinking from a crystal clear stream, creek, river, or waterfall, you never know if a dead animal or other contaminant is upstream, and that can get into your water. Getting sick in a survival situation is a sure way to put your survival at-risk, so you want to avoid it as much as possible. Always treat *all* water, but be particularly careful in treating water sourced from still bodies of water. You should treat water with proper filters designed for hikers; however, you can boil the water for 20 minutes over a fire if you do not have access to filters.

Fire

Fire is essential for survival because it provides two benefits: heat and a cooking source. You can also use the fire to sterilize things either through the smoke or through boiling water to clean off equipment such as stainless steel cookware. If you are in an urban setting and continue to have access to power, you will replace fire with electricity. If not, however, you will switch it out for fire.

In an urban environment, you may have the capacity to have a fire in your own home if you have a fireplace. Keep wood nearby and have plenty of starting materials and combustion tools on hand so you can start and maintain fire as needed. Lint out of your dryer is excellent for an urban starting material, as is cotton, cardboard tubes, and tissue papers. If you have a gas fireplace, check for leakages in the fuel line before using it, as some emergencies can damage the leak, and the gas from your fireplace is deadly. As well, gas fireplaces will not work as a cooking source, so you will need access to something else to cook your food with.

If you do not have a fireplace in your house, your next order of business is to look for a grill. Barbecues will provide a source of heat when outdoors, as well as a means for cooking. If you do not have access to a barbecue, you should build a firepit safely away from your building, but close enough that you can use it for heat and cooking. For the inside of your house, candles work as a light source and provide a small source of heat if you have enough candles or large enough candles. For warmth, bundle up on extra bedding and clothes if it happens to be a cold night. Standing out next to your fire with thick clothes and a blanket can help heat them, so you are likely to stay warm throughout the entire night. You can also sleep skin-to-skin alongside other humans if it is unusually cold to protect your core temperature and help keep you alive.

In a natural environment, a fire will provide a means of heat, an opportunity for you to keep yourself clean, and a spot for you to cook. Your heating fire should be kept near your camp. In contrast, your cooking fire and food should be at least 100 yards away from where you are sleeping to avoid attracting wildlife directly to your sleeping quarters. This way, if wildlife comes across your food, and they will, they do not come across you at the same time.

Creating a fire in the woods requires a certain amount of skill as you have to know how to build a fire so it will start, how to light your fire, and how to maintain it without accidentally smothering it. To thrive, fires rely on what is called the triangle of fire, which means they need oxygen, fuel, and heat. With these three elements, your fire will thrive, and without them, it will either go out or fail to get started in the first place.

There are two fire lays you can use that will help you get started, though I go over three additional ones in *Survival 101: Bushcraft*. These two fire lays are called the teepee fire, and the log cabin fire. A teepee fire is best for heat, while a log cabin fire is best for cooking.

Before you can light a fire, you are going to need what is known as a tinder bird nest, which is a starter for any fire. A tinder bird nest uses starting materials such as dry grass, twigs, cotton, dried pine cones, dried tree bark, and the lichen known as old man's beard. You want to take all of these materials and form a small birds nest shape using them, as this will give you plenty of starting materials to get your fire going. The idea with any fire is to get the tinder burning first, then the kindling, and then the actual fuel logs. From there, you can continue to add logs to your already burning fire to keep it going.

The teepee fire lay is created by taking a bird's nest and placing it in the center of where you want your fire to be. Then, use kindling to form a teepee shape over the tinder. You will continue doing this until you have used pencil-sized twigs. Then you will create a more massive teepee around your kindling structure using actual logs, which will be the fuel for your fire. After you have created this structure, you can light the tinder on the innermost part of your teepee, and that fire will reach up to burn your kindling, then your fuel logs. From there, you will have a roaring fire.

A log cabin style fire lay is created by interlocking logs to create a cabin style fire lay. To create your log cabin fire lay, you are going to use smaller pieces of wood, not much larger than tinder. You will lay two pieces of wood parallel to each other on the ground and far enough apart to create a space between them but close enough that when you lay more kindling across them, the second layer of kindling comfortably rests with either end on the previous kindling. Your second layer of kindling should be laid out as two pieces of kindling crossing over the ends of the first layer, creating a square shape. Continue layering kindling in either direction until you have about 5-8 layers. You want enough there to start a reasonable fire, but not so much that it takes a while to burn. The goal with a log cabin fire lay is that it burns down quickly so that you can cook on a low fire and the embers at the base of the fire. You can start your log cabin fire lay by placing a tinder bird nest in the center and lighting the fire, which will then catch the wood on fire. Make sure your bird nest is large enough to reach the fire you have laid around it. You can always tighten the inner square by placing the logs closer together if need be.

Food

If you have enough time left on your day of arrival, you will want to go in search of food right away. Ideally, you should have at least a couple of hours left before nightfall to avoid being caught away from camp in the dark. If you do not have someone who can stay at the camp and monitor the fire while you go in search of food, you are going to want to wait on building your fire until you return. If you do not have enough time before nightfall, you will make your fire right away, sleep through the night, then start on finding food first thing in the morning.

In an urban environment, you want to account for your food by having at least two weeks' worth of food in your pantry at all times. Once you have two weeks' worth of food stored, you want to move on to storing enough food for a few months or up to a year. It may sound like a lot, but the reality is that you never know how much you will need. Having more than enough is always better than having none at all.

If you are in an urban environment and an emergency strikes and you have not yet stored everything you need, you are going to need to find a way to source food. The first and possibly most obvious means of searching is to look in local grocery stores and markets for food. If the stores have not shut down, prioritize buying sale items of non-perishable ready to eat foods. This way, you can buy enough for the foreseeable future. If the emergency you are facing has shut down or diminished grocery stores, you can look to nearby towns for farmers who may have what you need. In many emergencies, charitable organizations will rapidly come through and offer food and water to those who have been affected. However, there is always a chance that this does not work out for you. For example, if you are not located or if they run out of resources, you will need to rely on yourself for your food and water. If it comes to it, you can look to hunt and forage your foods using the same means that natural survivalists will need to do. Be extremely cautious when foraging or trapping food in urban environments to avoid breaking laws or accidentally injuring someone else, or becoming injured in the process. Avoid using dangerous weapons in favor of trapping, fishing, and foraging, which are all much safer means of gathering food in an urban environment. They do not pose a threat to other humans in the area.

Sourcing food in a natural environment is a large undertaking. Learning to forage, fish, and trap is the best way to get started. Foraging is perhaps the easiest undertaking when it comes to acquiring food, as you only need to source the food, you do not need to do much to prepare it. In the wilderness, there are hundreds of plants that are healthy for you to eat, and there are hundreds more that are dangerous for you to eat. The only safe way to know what is available for you is to find a book on local foraging or take a local foraging class to discover what to look for, how to harvest the foraging items, and how to consume them safely. Many times, you can find herbalists who offer plant walks that will educate you on how to safely forage food in your local area. They can answer any questions you may have when it comes to safely sourcing food in the wilderness.

Fishing and trapping are slightly more challenging as you have to prepare the food you find, both through gutting it and through cooking it properly to avoid becoming sick. It is advised that upon leaving an urban environment, you bring fishing line and hooks with you, as well as snare wires for trapping. With your fishing lines and hooks, you will want to tie the line along the end of a sturdy stick and make it long enough that you can dangle it out in the water. Then, you will tie your hook on the other end and attach a piece of bait to it. A small bug like a worm or a caterpillar will work perfectly. Look for an area of water where it is relatively still, such as an inlet on a river or a deeper, slower-moving part of a creek. Then, dangle your line! You might need to bob it in and out a few times to encourage fish to bite, but soon enough, someone will bite. If not, see if you can find a similar area that may be more densely populated.

To prepare a fish for eating, you will rub the back of your knife along the flesh of the fish to remove the scales. Then, you will start at the tail end of the fish by inserting your knife in to make an incision. Make your incision deep enough that it goes into the middle of the fish, but not so deep that you completely cut the fish in half. Remove the innards and gills from the fish with your hand, then chop off the head and tail. Rinse it off and cook it thoroughly so that it is safe for eating.

Snares are set by tying a noose into snare wire and placing a snare somewhere that small to medium game animals are likely to frequent. Then, you mostly wait for one to trap itself and die in the snare. The most popular game to attract in snares are rabbits and hares, though you might also use snares to capture squirrels, rats, or other rodents.

Creating your snare noose will require you first to create the noose itself. Snare wire will work best for this, but twisted copper from inside small appliance power cords, picture hanging wire, craft wire, and headphone wire work, too. You will start your snare by creating a loop on one end of the wire. With wire, you will make a loop at twist the wire several times over to make sure the loop is strong enough, as you do not want it to break when the animal begins to struggle. Otherwise, you will lose the animal. Next, you are going to thread the other end of the wire through the loop you have made. The loop should be able to freely move up and down the wire, as this is how it will tighten when an animal begins to run or struggle inside of the snare.

You want to set your snare with the leader line, or the end of the snare that is not actively contributing to the noose loop, tied tightly to a branch or a part of brush that will not break under the pressure of the snare being activated by the animal. Then, the noose itself should be set open, ideally hooked around a small twig or something near the ground to keep the snare open and in place. When an animal runs through the snare, it will tighten, effectively trapping the animal.

Once you have trapped a small animal, you need to process it. You will need rope to hang the animal, heavy-duty scissors and two knives: a smaller one for precision cutting, and a larger one for cutting through joints. You will need a container for the rabbit parts you will keep and one for the parts you won't want. The container for the parts you will keep should have cold, filtered water in it. The other one should be easy enough to transport the discarded animal parts far away from your camp to avoid attracting any wild animals in your direction.

You will start by hanging the animal with rope by their back legs over a low hanging branch, which will make it easy for you to access the animal and process it. For a rabbit, you will cut the head and two front feet off so it can bleed out through the feet. For anything else, you can sever the arteries and veins in their throat. Once the bleeding stops, you will cut around the back legs down to the meat layer using a small precision knife. Then, you will pull the hide off of the animal. You may need to use the knife to carefully cut the pelt away from the skin at some points, but gently tugging it off should work for the most part. You will also cut from the inner thigh across to the bellybutton so that as you pull the pelt off the genital area remains covered in hair. Go to the back of the rabbit and do the same thing, leaving fur around the anus and tail area. At this point, the pelt should easily slide off since the front feet and head are not in place to stop the hide from moving. With rabbits and hares, you can cut the pelt so that it hangs flat and dry it out to be used for future projects if you will be surviving long term. These pelts are excellent for warming up the insides of shelters, sewing together to create warm clothing, and using for other similar purposes.

If you are cooking a small animal like a squirrel, you will not remove the limbs. You will only gut the animal. If you are preparing a larger animal like a rabbit or a hare, you will start by removing the front legs from the animal and placing them in your meat bucket. Use your larger, sturdier knife to severe the ligaments and pry the leg from the body. Next, take your knife and run it down the backbone from the tail to the clavicle bone. You want the cut about as deep as the animal's ribs; then, you will cut this back strip out by tracing the shape just under the ribs. This will give you two pieces of back meat.

Next, you will turn the animal around and start to harvest the organs. Since the lower portions of the animal are removed already, this part is more straightforward. A ruptured organ will require you to discard any meat contaminated by the fluids from that ruptured organ, so you need to be careful. At least this way, you have about four useful pieces of meat already off the animal if you make a mistake. You will start by cutting a small hole into the stomach lining, taking care to only go through the skin layer. Then, you will insert a finger into the hole press the inner organs away from the stomach lining so that you can carefully cut the lining open. You will then use your hands to pull the organs out of the meat. While you can eat the heart and liver, you do not have to. You can discard these if you prefer not to. Simply tug the organs out and away from the animal with a firm tug, and they should all come out safely without rupturing. Throw them away. Finally, remove the hind legs of the animal, then toss the tail and lower spinal portion into your discard bin. Now you are done!

You will want to properly wash your harvested meat, and safely discard the rest of it far away from your camp. Properly wash everything that you used to harvest the animal, too, to avoid any animals tracking you by the scent of the animal you harvested.

You should always cook game meat and fish well beyond what you would cook at home, as it has been wildly harvested, and may have bacteria or parasites growing in it. For game meat, always char the outsides and cook it until the insides are nearly dry. This way, you properly kill any bacteria or parasites that may be lingering in the meat, and that has the potential to make you sick.

Store your meat in proper containers at least 100 yards away from camp. The safest way to do so is to wrap them up in a tarp and hang them out from a branch where they will be too high to be grabbed from the ground and too low to be seized from the branch. This way, no animals can steal your harvested food. Make sure the meat is stored properly in ample amounts of salt, as this prevents it from developing bacteria while you store it. If you cannot adequately store your food, only harvest what you can eat in a few hours on a day to day basis.

Safety

Securing your safety in a survival setting is of utmost importance. Exposure, wildlife, natural disasters, illness, injury, and possible ambush from other humans are all things to consider in various survival circumstances. You can protect yourself by maintaining proper hygiene, and by being prepared to defend yourself in case of an attack. Otherwise, you can protect yourself by steering clear of areas where natural disasters are likely to occur and having a proper shelter in place for you to protect yourself from exposure.

In an urban setting, protecting yourself is reasonably easy because you have access to an abundance of homes to protect you from such things. The main things you will need to look for are leaks, contamination, bacteria, and attacks from the outside world. Gas leaks, pipe leaks, down powerlines feeding live electricity into the ground, and contaminated water, are all common risks when a natural disaster has struck. You need to immediately look for and be aware of any of these things happening so you can protect yourself adequately. Bacteria can come into the house or can grow in the house from inadequate practices such as improper food storage or removal of refuse. Maintaining proper hygiene is imperative to avoid having bacteria build-up and creating a hazard in your life.

If you are in a situation where other humans could harm you, you need to be prepared to protect yourself. Weaponry such as guns, knives, and bows should be considered. Bars on your windows and proper locks on your doors can also protect you from people trying to break in.

In a natural environment, you need to protect yourself from exposure, wildlife, widowmakers, and illness or injury. You can do this with adequate shelter, fire, and proper clothes to keep yourself warm and dry. Having defensive weaponry on hand is essential in case an animal comes through your camp. Protecting yourself by keeping all food sources and scents far away from camp is important, too. You should always change out of the clothes you have cooked and eaten in and leave them at your cooking camp 100 yards away, so you do not accidentally bring the smell back to your sleeping camp with you. Staying away from common areas where animals hang out is ideal, too, as it keeps you protected from the animals who may be passing by. With widowmakers, you already know to avoid them when you are setting up camp. However, you should also be prepared to avoid them when you are traveling, especially if there is wind, rain, or snow. These can encourage dead trees to fall and can injure or kill you while you are away from camp. Prevent injuries by wearing proper footwear, walking on firm ground, moving intentionally and slowly, and protecting your skin from cuts and scrapes. Even one tiny scratch can become infected and lead to death in the wilderness, so avoid them at all costs.

In addition to preventing injury, you also need to prevent illness by maintaining proper core temperature, keeping yourself warm and dry. Promptly care for any wounds you sustain by keeping them clean and dry. You should also properly cleanse any food and water you are going to eat or drink, hang your bedding and clothes in the sun for the sun to sterilize them, and bathe yourself in campfire smoke, which can sterilize any bacteria that may be on your body.

These are all essential ways of keeping up hygiene so you do not end up sick, which can quickly become a deadly situation in the wilderness.

CHAPTER 4
The Task Lists

Survival situations are not straightforward or simple. There are many tasks to secure your survival. There are 34 tasks to do if you are going to survive any situation you happen upon. Some of these tasks will need to be completed in advance, while others will need to be completed or finished in the event of an emergency. You will want to run through it in full, first, to prepare yourself, then run through it again in a survival setting to ensure that everything has been adequately completed. In this chapter, we will address the order and importance of each of these 34 tasks. In *Chapter 5: The 34 Tasks of Survival*, we will cover exactly how to fulfill each of these tasks.

Tasks 1 to 3: Preparing

The first three tasks on the task list are all about preparation. These two tasks can and should be done well in advance of anything going wrong, and should be stored in an area where they are easily accessible for mild, moderate, and extreme emergencies.

Although preparing may seem like a small, unimportant task, it is essential to understand that preparation is imperative to your success in a survival situation. During a period where no threats are looming, preparing for survival is easy. At this point, you can access everything you would need in an emergency, place it together in an easily-accessible location, and ensure it is ready for a possible emergency to strike.

People often make the mistake of pretending they have all the time in the world to prepare, which results in procrastination and a failure to ever truly prepare. As a result, when an emergency strikes, they find themselves lacking everything they need. During those scary moments when time is of the essence, they either do not have the time to access essential emergency preparedness items, or the supplies have sold out, such as with the pandemic of 2020. Waiting is often a dangerous game that can lead to an emergency becoming worse than it needs to be, or possibly leading to fatalities because essential preparedness items were not available.

The moral of the story is, do not wait until an emergency to prepare yourself. Assume that an emergency is coming at the least expected of moments, because they can and will, and prepare yourself accordingly. Ensure you are always prepared so that if you ever need your preparedness items, you are ready to go. It is better to be overprepared rather than underprepared in a true emergency.

Tasks 4 to 5: Assessing

Tasks four and five require you to assess the area of the emergency, and each person involved in your survival team. In mild emergencies, a quick area check involves checking the status of everyone involved in the emergency. In extreme settings, this could include checking everyone's abilities and needs, as well as their overall physical condition so that you know who can do what, and what needs have to be considered for survival. Environmentally, you want to check the area to ensure that you know where your essentials can be found.

During an emergency, it may seem impossible or unreasonable to assess the situation. Your emotions may have you wanting to dive right in and immediately get to work, especially if the emergency is dire and time is of the essence. Failure to assess an emergency before jumping into the situation can lead to a far greater emergency than you initially started with. For example, if someone has fallen down a cliff and is sitting at the bottom, injured, attempting to scale the cliff yourself could lead to you also being injured. Neither of you being able to call for help. Although your instinct may tell you to immediately rescue that person, the better idea is to ensure you have adequate help and resources to help that person safely. This way, you do not end up with a larger and more damaging emergency.

Assessment in an emergency survival situation should include assessing yourself and the individuals you are partaking in the survival situation with. Especially if you will be required to survive in the woods for any period of time, you need to know what everyone is capable of and what everyone's limits are. Failure to adequately assess capabilities and limits could lead to a lack of resources being acquired due to someone being incapable, or someone finding themselves facing a medical emergency due to pushing their limits too hard. Although survival situations are trying and limits will inevitably be pushed, you should avoid pushing them too far as this can lead to tragic circumstances and unnecessary illness, injury, or even death.

Tasks 6 to 12: Prevention

Prevention and prevention checklists are used to ensure that everything is kept safe when you are in a survival setting. This includes preventing firearm injuries, fires, drowning, and poisoning. You also need to assess the environment to be aware of and prevent damage from environmental threats, and those that could be caused by man-made threats. In addition to environmental threats, you need to prevent anyone from being injured or falling ill due to improper practices.

Understand that adequate prevention will come in the form of practical measures taken to avoid illness or injury, as well as adequate education on situations that could lead to potential illness or injury. For example, with firearms, sufficient measures such as using the safety or keeping inactive firearms in a locked safe are essential as a practical means of preventing accidental injury or death. Likewise, adequate education on behalf of anyone who might be using the firearm can prevent accidental injury or death caused by improper usage of a dangerous weapon.

As with preparation, ensure that these measures are met ahead of time. Any prevention measures that involve an educational aspect to ensure total prevention is achieved should be learned before a survival situation arises. This ensures that in the heat of a stressful and often scary situation, you are not pressured to attempt to learn new information. During times of high stress, the human mind is not typically capable of absorbing new information, which means that there is a higher risk of mistakes occurring, and therefore illness, injury, or even death could occur.

Should you plan on surviving with other people outside of your household, ensure that they also take prevention seriously. In some cases, such as with foodborne illnesses or improper firearm use, another person's improper education and prevention could lead to yours or someone else's accidentally illness, injury, or death. Ensuring that everyone is properly educated and capable of following essential security measures is the only way to guarantee near-perfect prevention measures are applied in a dangerous situation.

Tasks 13 to 14: Communication

Communication must be secured between the A-Team and, if possible, the outside world. This can be done by securing an emergency radio and ensuring someone is available to listen to it at all times. It can also be done by creating a code word list which will be used by the A-Team to identify certain situations. This, in a sense, is used as your own language so that the A-Team can communicate quickly and promptly.

An essential step in securing communication involves understanding the psychology of an individual during an emergency situation. Recognize that high stress can reduce the quality of communication, creating a higher instance for arguments, as well as miscommunications that could lead to dangerous situations. Accommodate for this by frequently discussing communication measures that will be taken in an emergency situation to minimize miscommunications and avoid arguments.

It may also be beneficial to discuss how each member of the A-Team navigates stress. Understanding each other's tendencies during stressful situations ensures that instinctive stress responses in each individual are not taken personally by other members of the camp. This is a great preventative measure applied to communication that is intended to support each member of the camp and improve the quality of camp life, while also minimizing accidents triggered by miscommunications or misunderstandings. It also boosts camp morale by keeping everyone on the same page, which, believe it or not, is an essential means of survival. A miserable camp makes it hard for people to feel committed to survival because it may seem like there is no point, or they are not gaining anything valuable by living through the emergency. Positive camp morale encourages everyone to keep going for the sake of each other and their own wellbeing.

Tasks 15 to 25: The First Five

The first five, including water, shelter, fire, food, and safety, are essential to your survival, so you are going to need to address and secure the first five for the entire A-Team. You will prepare for the first five ahead of time by setting up measures to protect your A-Team from mild to extreme situations. Then, in active survivalist situations, you will invoke the terms of those measures to ensure that you are actively taking action to secure the first five and survive amid a crisis.

Realize that once you find yourself in an emergency where survival must be secured, this is where you *start.* Ideally, all of your preparedness, assessments, prevention, and communication should be sorted out by now. The only step you may take from previous tasks would be to re-assess the situation based on the present emergency you are facing. This ensures that your A-Team assessments are recent and relevant, you are aware of the state of your current BOHS location, and you are all able to coordinate an effective plan to secure the first five. These initial assessments should be relevant *only* to the securing of the first five. After those have been secured, you can conduct deeper assessments to ensure long-term survival, if that is required.

If you have a particularly large A-Team, or if you have members of the A-Team with special requirements, please ensure that you create a game plan ahead of time. While a survival game plan involving who would do what is important, it is especially important for those who need to secure a large amount of equipment, or may be dealing with special requirements that make securing equipment more challenging. Having a general game plan in advance means you only have to modify that game plan, rather than start from scratch. This saves precious time and ensures you are much quicker and more effective at gathering necessary supplies for survival.

Tasks 26 to 27: Special Equipment

Special equipment is required for most modern humans, and that equipment must be accessed and secured. Keeping individual documents on a thumb drive and a cloud drive, as well as having emergency equipment available for work and/or school, is important. You will need to have all of this organized and set up at all times.

During a dire emergency, special equipment may not seem important. You may think that your work-related or school-related information is irrelevant and that the pressing issue is your survival. Of course, this is true to an extent. Your number one focus should be securing your survival, and the more pressing the emergency, the less likely you will be able to secure these aspects of your survival. However, it is essential to remember that emergencies do eventually end, and society will strive to get back to normal. Attempting to recover your work-related and school-related items, as well as special documents like ID and other necessities, will be much more challenging in a post-emergency situation. This can also elongate your stress and make emotionally recovering from an emergency even more challenging than it already is. Try to remember that life will continue after the emergency, and prepare yourself for that.

Task 28 to 31: Equipment Checklists

Aside from personal equipment, you need your survival equipment. This includes equipment for travel, for your survival vest, for yourself, and your car. You want to have a checklist that defines all of the items required, as well as all of the items on the checklist available in each area and organized at any given time. You should frequently check to make sure everything is there and in stock, that it is in proper working order, and that it has not expired.

Checklists may seem like small, unnecessary aspects of survival. Still, they are essential tools that can make all the difference. A properly-populated checklist serves to remind you of all the items that are essential to survival. Understand that it is nearly impossible to know what you will need in an emergency until you are in one and realize you do not have what you need. Fortunately, enough emergencies have happened by now that other people have recalled their needs and placed them together on well-populated lists served to protect you and your family from lacking an essential item during an emergency. Following these checklists ensures that you have everything you need.

During an active emergency, after you have secured your first five, you may review checklists to ensure you have everything required for short-term and long-term survival situations. This way, if you realize you are missing anything, you can improvise with bush-made tools or other resources so that when that item comes up as needed, you are ready with an alternative.

Tasks 32 to 34: Leaving

The final tasks are relevant to leaving and include having everything pre-packaged and ready to go. This will include having a checklist for GnG Bags that are developed for mild situations, as well as GnG Bags that are developed for moderate to extreme situations. Both bags should always be fully stocked and ready for use, no matter what.

It is essential that you keep all of your survival and emergency equipment prepared inside of GnG bags from the start. Storing them loosely in a closet, garage, or shed may result in you being unable to bring all or any items with you because they were not ready for immediate evacuation. In situations like hurricanes, fires, or earthquakes, immediate evacuation may be required to protect yourself from danger. Ready-packed bags prevents you from having to make the hard choice of risking injury or death or leaving your preparedness items behind during an emergency.

Ensure that you efficiently pack your bags and that you practice carrying them away from the house. It would be incredibly disappointing to realize that your well-packed bags were packed too heavy, or in such a way that makes them impossible to fit into your vehicle upon evacuation. A proper practice run ensures that everything can be reasonably removed from your home and brought with you in a GnG situation.

CHAPTER 5
The 34 Tasks Of Survival

The 34 tasks of survival are done in two phases. The first phase is for you to run through all of these tasks *before* finding yourself in a survival situation so that you are confident that you are prepared for anything that may happen. The second phase is to run through them during an emergency to ensure you are ready to survive that emergency. In moderate to extreme emergencies, you will likely find that there is first the next phase of survival, which is to protect yourself against whatever is coming. That may not be entirely possible for you to plan, as you cannot anticipate when a crisis will strike, so you are going to have to think on your toes and do what is right at that moment. For example, in an earthquake, it would not be wise to immediately run back to your IRP or ERP and begin executing your tasks. Instead, you will first need to survive the earthquake; then, you will need to start taking action on the immediate follow-up. Since there is no way to prepare for exactly what you will do in the very moment crisis strikes, you need to educate yourself and trust in your skill when it comes to surviving that initial strike. Immediately after the initial crisis has struck, however, you need to jump into action with your survival plan.

Ensure that you complete each task entirely before moving on to the next one. As well, learn how to execute the task or use any relevant tools in case of an emergency. For example, task 28 reflects travel equipment. You need to know how to collect and store your travel equipment, as well as how to use it so that when you need it, you are familiar with how it works. Practice runs should be performed with your A-Team, too, to ensure you are all on the same page.

It would be wise to keep a copy of this task list available in a printed format in your GnG Bag, as well so that when you get into the bush, you can look through it and refresh yourself. Sometimes, no matter how well you educate yourself, a state of emergency can prevent your memory from functioning correctly, and having vital information written down can support you with recalling everything that needs to be done.

Task 1: A-Team Contacts

Having a contact sheet on hand is crucial when it comes to survival. You want your A-Team Contacts list to include contact information for every person on your A-Team, including yourself, as well as important numbers to know. This includes the numbers for doctors and specialists for each member of the A-Team, poison control numbers, emergency contact numbers, work and school numbers, and insurance and personal identification numbers. These numbers ensure that anyone can immediately be contacted in case of an emergency. Every member of the A-Team should have a copy. You should also have one in your GnG bags so that they can be accessed quickly when you are away from home.

Task 2: Water Bottles

Even in a short term emergency, you are going to need to have water available to sustain yourself. A lack of access to water can rapidly become an emergency in and of itself. You should have two quarts of water per person in your house, which would create enough water for six days for each person. The water should be kept clean, filtered, and stored in a way that is easy to access and easy to transport. While canned water kept in glass canning jars may last longer than those kept in plastic, keep in mind the glass adds weight when it comes to transporting.

Stainless steel canteens are a great alternative to glass as they remain sterile, will not leach chemicals into the water, and are much more lightweight when transporting. Plus, canteens can be worn around your neck, which can free up space inside of the GnG bag.

Task 3: First Aid Kit

A well-stocked first-aid kit should be essential for any household. They are useful for treating everyday injuries at home, and they can be lifesaving in certain emergency situations. Stock your first aid kit with standard first aid items, as well as items unique to your family's medical needs. If you know that a certain family member is prone to something, in particular, stock up on extra supplies for that particular ailment. For example, if a family member is prone to excessive bleeding, keep additional gauze and bandages on hand in case they sustain an injury.

Every first aid kit should have:

- Emergency phone numbers and important personal contacts
- Safety pins
- Tweezers
- Scissors
- Instant ice packs
- Latex gloves (disposable) or neoprene gloves if you have a latex allergy
- Flashlight with extra batteries that are stored in a separate bag
- Sterile gauze pads in small and large squares for dressing wounds
- Self-adhesive tape and adhesive medical tape
- Roller bandages and triangle bandages for keeping injured limbs in place
- Adhesive bandages in an assortment of sizes

- Antiseptic wipes and soap
- Pencil and paper
- Thermometer
- Pocket mask or face shield
- CPR mask
- Emergency blanket
- Eye patches
- Coins for a payphone and cash in small bills
- Drugs like ibuprofen, naproxen, and acetaminophen for pain, and diphenhydramine for minor allergic reactions
- Medications that are unique to the people the first aid kit will be serving, such as specific drugs, inhalers, epi-pens, insulin, and other necessary supplies
- A first aid manual

If you have a family member who is prone to bleeding, or if you are going into an area where lacerations could occur, and you will not have access to immediate medical support, you may also keep a diaper or a few feminine pads in your first aid kit. These are made of clean, absorbent material that can absorb a large amount of blood without having to be removed. This means you can apply consistent pressure for longer with them.

Task 4: Check Status of A-Team

The fourth task for survival is to check the status of your A-Team. If you are in the preparation phase, you will pay attention to more long term and average conditions. At the same time, if you are in survival mode, you will check for more recent, present, and pressing issues.

During the preparation phase, you should compile a "profile" of each member of the A-Team. This profile should include that person's age, date of birth, and overall health. Consider overall physical condition, including their weight and strength, as well as how easy it is (or isn't) for them to perform more physical tasks such as walking or running. Also, take note of their medical status, any allergies they may have, and any medications they may be on. Consider any special needs they may have, as well as their ability to engage in specific tasks that are related to survival such as swimming, driving, splitting wood, carrying things, and so forth. Lastly, consider what type of access they have to vehicles.

You should prepare your survival plan to ensure that each member of the A-Team's needs will be met accordingly. As well, plan for plenty of room for necessities to be packed, and consider their abilities and needs when locating your BOHS and delegating duties. Make sure any tasks delegated to each member of the A-Team are duties they can reasonably handle and allow them to maintain those duties.

Review all status profiles and designations of each A-Team member before engaging in any survival situation. You need to know that you have up-to-date information on their health, wellness, energy, abilities, and needs. You also need to be confident that any tasks delegated to this individual are tasks that they will reasonably be able to assume and complete while you are in a survivalist situation. While everyone needs to pull their weight, your survival camp will run best if everyone is tasked with something that is within their ability as it ensures that the job will get done right and that there will be minimal chance of running into injuries or illnesses along the way.

Task 5: Area Study

An area study happens over three parts, and it will be used to help your A-Team prepare a plan for survival. The first part of the task is to study your general geography, the second part of the task is to study your BOHS location, and the third part of the task is to review the area of the BOHS location once you arrive in a survival situation.

Studying your general geography is important as it allows you to know what to expect in the area where you will be surviving. This study should include a study of the landscape, vegetation, animals, and likely threats in your area. Keep yourself updated and knowledgeable in these things so you can use it to your advantage in any survival situation. You must expand your studies to your entire geographical location and not just the area of your BOHS, as you never know when an emergency could make your BOHS inaccessible or unusable. This way, if your BOHS fails, you can find an alternative and still feel confident surviving in that area.

Studying your BOHS location before a real emergency hits is a good idea as it allows you to understand the geography immediately surrounding the BOHS. During this study, you want to locate everything you learned from your general geography study of your area and use that to your advantage. Find water, the best areas for trapping, and the best locations for shelter.

Reviewing your BOHS location in a survival situation only requires a mild area study. At this point, you already know the region quite well based on your previous studies, so you simply need an updated view on what is going on and what the best methods for navigation and survival would be in this area. This allows you to recognize any changes that may have occurred, refresh yourself on anything you learned previously, and ultimately familiarize yourself with the area. It will be a lot easier for you to survive in a familiar setting than it will for you to survive in a foreign one, so take this task seriously. In a familiar setting, you are aware of what is normal. Therefore it becomes easier to spot abnormalities or potential threats caused by the geography or the local wildlife. In a foreign setting, you are not entirely aware of what to expect, and therefore it becomes more challenging to spot normal from abnormal and to protect yourself against geography and wildlife.

Task 6: Firearm Prevention

Firearms are imperative to survival situations, especially ones where you will be residing in the bush. A gun will protect you against wildlife and intruders and keep you safe from anything that may be going on in your area. With that being said, guns must be used and stored safely to prevent any accidental injuries or deaths from occurring. Every single gun should have a safety on it. That safety should be secured in place anytime the gun is not actively being used. This safety should be applied when the gun is being stored, as well as when it is being carried.

Your day to day dwelling, as well as your BOHS, should both have locations for you to safely store your guns so that they are inaccessible to anyone but yourself or those who have the code to your safe. Keeping your guns in these safes anytime they are not in use is crucial to avoid accidental injury or death.

The next method of prevention you need to consider with guns is preventing injury or death by teaching everyone how to use them safely. Knowing how to safely use a gun prevents direct injury from the gun itself or injury from a failure to use the gun for protection. To put it simply, if you cannot aim and stop the attacker, you will end up being attacked. Everyone on the A-Team should learn how to safely load, aim, and shoot a gun, as well as what to do with the gun after. Target practice is also a good idea and should be completed at least once per week at the camp during a survival situation to ensure that everyone has a strong aim and is able to safely protect themselves in case of an emergency.

Task 7: Fire Prevention

Fire prevention needs to be practiced at home, as well as at your survival site. Fire prevention at home can be accomplished with smoke alarms, escape routes, and fire extinguishers. You should also be sure not to leave any small appliances plugged in or left on, especially when you are away from home. As well, keep flammable materials away from heat sources and open flames, and do your part in preventing fires.

At camp, fire prevention can be accomplished by keeping fires properly contained and safely away from fuel sources. They should also be kept away from low hanging branches, dry brush, and your shelter, as a fire can quickly jump over and start burning everything around it. Every single fire should be put out when it is not being monitored or in use, to ensure that it is not able to cause uncontrolled burning. Take extra precautions when lighting a fire to keep you warm through the night. Keep the area free of debris, carefully block it with rocks to prevent it blowing out of the fire pit, and stay far enough away that it does not accidentally catch your sleeping bag or supplies on fire.

Should a fire break out, you will need something on hand to help put it out. At home, flour and fire extinguishers are great. In the bush, dirt and water are great. Flour or dirt should be used on grease and alcohol fires, as water will only worsen the fire. On all other fires, fire extinguishers and water are fine. If you do not know what caused the fire, use something to smother it, or get far away from the fire as quickly as possible. If you are at home, call for help. If you are in the bush and not presently afraid of the authorities, you should call for help in that scenario, too. Keep the emergency numbers for fire on hand at all times so that you can quickly call if needed.

Task 8: Drowning Prevention

Drowning is a serious risk for death, whether you realize it or not. An average of 332 people die per year from accidental drownings. While that may not seem like much, the risk is drastically increased if the person is particularly young, or if they are unfit and in an emergency situation. At home, youths, particularly toddlers and younger, are at highest risk for drowning. Elders or those who may have a condition such as narcolepsy can be high at risk, too, if they take a bath and find themselves suddenly submerged and unable to get out. Weak swimmers are especially endangered in survival situations where you may need to survive near large bodies of water or rapidly moving rivers.

At home, drowning prevention can be accomplished by avoiding allowing anyone who is particularly young, elderly, or ill with certain conditions to be around bodies of water without supervision or proper safety measures in place. The young should always be supervised, period. Those who are elderly or who have medical conditions can be protected by having proper seats installed in their tubs and rails to make getting in and out much easier.

In a survival situation, you must be prepared to look for all possible risks of drowning and then prevent them in whatever ways possible. If anyone on the A-Team is not a strong swimmer, either avoid crossing water altogether, look for alternate routes, or look for shallow areas where they can walk across. Avoid camping out near any fast-moving, deep, or rough bodies of water. As well, avoid ever putting your back to the water when you are at the top of a cliff or bank on the body of dangerous waters, as one misstep could lead you right off the edge.

Task 9: Poison Prevention

Poison prevention is another prevention practice that needs to be done both at home and in camp. At home, the most common culprits for poisonings are cleaning supplies and contaminated water or foods. In the bush, poisoning commonly comes from what you drink or consume.

At home, always be extremely careful when dealing with chemicals, especially those that are in cleaning solutions. You must be cautious about exposure by minimizing or eliminating a cleaning solution's contact with your skin, eyes, and mouth. You should avoid ever consuming any, either purposefully or accidentally, such as by accidentally spraying food on the counter while you are cleaning and then later eating the food. You should avoid inhaling too many of the fumes. In some cases, you need to avoid inhaling any fumes, period. You also need to prevent anyone in your family, especially young kids who would not know better, from accessing these solutions to avoid accidental poisonings in children.

At home, *never* mix the following solutions as they can be fatal:

- Bleach and vinegar should never be mixed as they create chlorine gas, which, even at low levels, can cause respiratory damage.
- Bleach and ammonia should never be mixed as they create chloramine, which can also cause respiratory damage often to fatal degrees.
- Different drain cleaners (even from the same brand) should never be mixed because when they are combined can explode based on the chemicals in them. If you have recently treated a sink, do not treat it again later with a different product, instead call a plumber and let them know what you used.

- Hydrogen peroxide and vinegar may be mixed on surfaces but should never be stored mixed in the same container. Together, they create peracetic acid, which can be toxic and can irritate your eyes, skin, and respiratory system.
- Bleach and rubbing alcohol should never be mixed because they produce chloroform, which can be extremely irritating, toxic, and can cause you to pass out.

Be especially careful with cleaning products that are named after a brand and not the chemical within them. Not knowing what is in the cleaning solutions you are using can lead to you accidentally creating fatal mixes of chemicals. For example, many window cleaning solutions contain ammonia, so if you cleaned your windows and then immediately started cleaning a surface with bleach, you could create chloramine in the air, which could cause you to pass out. Anyone using household cleaners should always be old enough to do so, and knowledgeable enough to do so safely. Store them up high and locked away from anyone who should not be touching them.

At camp, you must be aware of poisonous plants, poisonous and venomous animals, and potential contaminants in water. Avoiding plants and animals and thoroughly filtering and purifying your water will prevent you from becoming endangered through either type of exposure. It is advised that you take time to identify local poison threats and keep a detailed list, with pictures if possible, laminated and present in your GnG bag so that when you reach your BOHS location, you have this available. That way, your list is relevant to your area and easy for you and everyone on the A-Team to understand and follow. Activated charcoal is always good to have on hand as you can pump someone's system to hopefully remove poison from someone's body, in case of accidental ingestion. If venomous animals are common in your area, learn the appropriate protocol to extract venom from bites. This way, any bites can be promptly treated.

Task 10: Environmental Danger Assessment and Prevention

Environmental dangers can be a severe threat to your wellbeing. In the bush, they are called widowmakers. You need to be prepared to assess for danger and prevent that risk from becoming a severe issue at any point so long as you are around it.

At home, you need to be aware of what your possible environmental dangers look like based on the geographical area that you live in, such as tornadoes, hurricanes, earthquakes, wildfires, or avalanches. While these threats are not going to occur every single day, they can develop rapidly. Knowing how to monitor for them will ensure that you are prepared if the threat of a natural disaster arises.

In the bush, you need to survey your survival area to identify any potential threats that may be present quickly. Avoid writing any threats off as being "unlikely" and instead honestly assess every possible danger right down to the last possible thing. Consider how you will prevent those dangers from harming anyone. Staying away from dangerous cliffs, monitoring possibly risky logs, and knowing how you will protect yourself and each other from local wildlife, will all keep you safe.

Task 11: Man-Made Danger Assessment and Prevention

The last assessment and prevention check that needs to be completed is the man-made danger assessment and prevention.

At home, man-made threats linger inside of your house in the form of natural gas lines, faulty wiring, poor building techniques, and other such issues. Outside, man-made threats can include dams, traffic, and even people bearing firearms in certain areas. You also want to be aware of things such as chemical plants, the government, or authoritarian figures who may be taking advantage of their authority, down electric wires, and even nearby drug houses where they may be cooking illegal drugs or chemicals. All of these types of threats can pose a threat to your safety and wellbeing, so they should be assessed, monitored, and addressed in terms of how you will prevent them from causing any direct threat to you, your family, or the A-Team. You should also have a plan for how you will proceed if the threat level increases.

In the bush, man-made dangers could include hydro dams or other man-made structures. These can be highly dangerous and should be avoided at all costs to avoid the looming threat. Other man-made dangers can be made from people right in your camp.

People swinging axes, carrying or shooting guns, fires, and even poorly designed building structures can be a risk. It is vital always to pause, assess any possible dangers of a situation beforehand, and proceed accordingly. Never use hazardous tools around other people without knowing where those other people are and knowing that they are aware of you using the device. Never carry, fell, or drop heavy items when you do not know where other people are. Be sure to double-check structures to ensure they are not at risk of falling or caving in. Also, make sure campfires are far enough away from the structure that you are not risking them being caught on fire.

Task 12: Map and Navigation Supplies

In an urban setting, relying on internet-based navigation systems or digital navigation systems is easy. You can turn them on through your cell phone or through devices that you set up in your car, or that are built into your car, and reliably follow them anywhere you need to go. In the bush, navigating is not quite so easy. Most internet-based or digital navigation systems will not work. If they do, they will eventually die and become unusable. You must have other means of navigation to protect yourself in the bush.

Navigation tools you should have include a detailed map of your destination, a compass, a pedometer, and markers you can use to mark your path. Ensure that you know how to use these tools and navigation techniques such as handrails, backstops, baselines, aiming off, and panic azimuths, so you can safely navigate your location. Each of these methods is described in *Survival 101: Bushcraft* and should be well-understood and used by everyone on the A-Team to ensure that everyone stays safe and easy to locate in the bush.

Task 13: Emergency Radio

Emergency radios are critical to have on hand and should be kept nearby at all times. Your emergency radio can be useful both at home and in the bush. A proper emergency radio should be one that can be powered by a hand crank. This ensures that if you run out of battery power or batteries, or if the battery compartment somehow becomes damaged, you can still charge the radio. One way radios and two-way radios are essential, depending on what emergency you are in.

One way radios are radios that allow people to listen to emergency messages through radio frequencies in the case of an event. They are frequently used by authorities to inform the public on looming and active threats such as storms or devastating earthquakes. Keeping your emergency radio on hand will allow you to hear live updates as the threat continues. Updates will often tell you what to do, how to stay safe, and when it is safe to come out of hiding.

Two-way radios are important in the bush as they can help you stay in contact with people who are in the bush with you. Be sure to get two-way radios that can be solar-powered and that have the most extended range possible. This way, they can be used from great distances, and you do not have to worry about charging the radios when you go out.

Task 14: A-Team Codewords

A-Team codewords are a benefit to have for two different reasons. First and foremost, code words can make talking to each other more efficient, and this can offer a range of benefits. In a dangerous situation, a single codeword is easier to say than an entire sentence, and it is easier to hear, too. For example, in a hospital, code blue means an adult is in cardiac arrest. Having a quick codeword indicates that you do not have to attempt to describe the situation through yelling or through a two-way radio, and people will be able to recognize the level of emergency and respond accordingly quickly. These codes can also be useful when hunting, as they can be whispered into radios or called to each other from a distance without alerting the animal to your presence. When hunting, short and quick codewords avoid alerting the animal, you are hunting that you are present. When hunting, there should be codewords used to indicate the presence of an animal and to indicate when someone is going to shoot an animal. This way, everyone knows where to look, and they can stay clear of the animal to avoid an accidental injury.

A-Team words are also helpful in situations where you may not necessarily trust the government or outsiders, and where outsiders may pose a threat. Like speaking in your language, code words can allow you to communicate specific information without outsiders knowing what you are talking about. If you are in a situation that is threatening and involves other people, this is a good way to avoid the others from knowing what you are talking about.

In some situations, you may not necessarily be able to talk out loud, but you may still need to communicate. Code signals or body languages, then, are excellent choices for these situations. In intimate settings, a particular finger or hand signal or even a signal with the face can send a particular piece of information. From distances, certain arm movements or leg movements or even poses with the entire body could convey certain pieces of information. Be sure that everyone on the A-Team knows exactly what the code words are and how to use them so that everyone is able to communicate clearly. As well, avoid creating too many and instead only use a necessary few. Review the code words regularly until everyone clearly remembers them in case of an emergency. This way, no one is left trying to recall what a certain code means or finds themselves misinterpreting it and exposing themselves to danger.

Task 15: Rotation and Inspection Checklist

To remain prepared for any emergency, you need to know that everything required for your survival is available at any given time. Being prepared means that you not only have everything put together and checklists are in place, but that you regularly go through these items to ensure that everything is still prepared for your survival in case of an emergency. This is one thing many beginner preppers forget to do, and what ends up happening is they find themselves in an emergency situation, only to realize that most of their gear has expired or is no longer in working order due to not having been used for so long. While it is great to know that you don't often need your survival gear, it would be a tragedy to need it and not have access to it because you have allowed it to expire or seize in storage.

Your rotation and inspection checklist should require you to periodically check through each of the 34 tasks to ensure that everything is prepared, and you know how to use it. You should also have a checklist that runs through all of the equipment you are to keep on hand so that you can go through it and check in on all of your gear, as well.

Every six months, you should go through your rotation and inspection checklists. Any food or consumable items that are coming up to expiry should be removed, used in everyday life, and promptly replaced with fresh materials. Thoroughly test all tools, items, and objects to ensure that all of the parts are working. Any broken gear should be removed from your kit and immediately replaced. *You are not done with the inspection until everything has been restored and in proper working order.* Be as prompt as you can about returning such things to avoid finding yourself in a situation where you have forgotten to return something and find yourself without it in an emergency situation.

Task 16: Water for Mild Emergency

Water for mild emergencies should be enough to last you up to 2 days. Bottled water works, though you need to be prepared to replace them every one to two years to prevent plastic from breaking down and contaminating your water. If you prefer, you can keep a 5-gallon jug on hand or even can your water in glass jars, which tends to last longer since glass will not break down into the water. You will, however, need to maintain canned water. Over the years, some of it will naturally disappear, so you may need to redo those jars to ensure that they are full.

Then, every 30 years, you are going to want to completely throw out all of the water and replace your cans lids, as they can start to rust, which can contaminate your water.

Two days of water for every person in your household, plus a bit extra is always ideal for mild emergencies. This way, if you find yourself in a situation where you cannot go out and get water, you have plenty of access. You will want to set aside 1 gallon of water per day, per person. You should also store enough for any pets in your household. This water needs to be safe enough to consume, but will also be used for other means such as brushing your teeth. So, let's say you have a family of four plus two dogs, you would need 6 gallons of water per day or 12 gallons of water for a two-day emergency.

Task 17: Water for Moderate to Extreme Emergency

For moderate to extreme emergencies, you need enough water for six days for everyone in your home. You will also need a means for filtering more water in case six days of water is not enough. Let's start by focusing on the six days of water for each person in your house. Again, you will need one gallon of water per day, per person, as well as water for your pets. So, if you are a family of four with two dogs, you would need six gallons of water per day or thirty-six gallons of water for six days. Thirty-six gallons of water would be 144 x 2-quart jars, or 7 x 5-gallon jugs plus a few water bottles to make up for the extra gallon. *Or* you could invest in water barrels. High-density polyethylene (HDPE) plastic water gallons are excellent for storing water in. One can store up to 55 gallons of water, which would exceed your daily usage needs by 19 gallons, or three extra days for a family of four humans and two pets. These extra days can be useful, so do not discredit this option just because it may be larger than your needs.

In addition to having extra water storage available, you should also have a means of filtering water. Toting 55-gallons of water into the bush would be virtually impossible, so you will want to fill your canteens out of the container and bring along as many canteens as you could reasonably carry. Then, you would have a filter or two available, which would allow you to clean your water in the bush. This way, you can fetch water from natural sources and purify it so that it is safe for you to consume or use on your body or in your cleaning rituals in the bush.

There are two types of filters you can use in the bush. Manual filters act like a strainer and allow you to pour your water through, and they purify your water in the process. Purifying drops or tablets are dropped into water, and they purify your water as they dissolve. You should have both available for an emergency so that you can clean your water for an extended period. Make sure you get filters that are intended for natural purposes, as standard filters that purify tap water will not suffice. Tap water has already been treated by water management crews in the city, which means your water filters for the faucet or the fridge further purify and essentially improve the flavor. Purifiers for natural water sources are much more advanced, and they can kill off all of the bacteria, viruses, and parasites that would typically be treated by water management crews in the city.

Task 18: Shelter for Mild Emergency

For a mild emergency, you want to make sure you have access to adequate shelter. Your house is plenty enough for shelter for a mild emergency; however, you should also have backup plans in case your shelter is not accessible or usable during the case of an emergency. With that, there are two levels of preparedness that need to occur for shelter for mild emergencies.

The first level is preparing your own home. It should be in proper working order and should be available for you to live in for up to two weeks without needing anything at any given time. You should have adequate clothes, bedding, cleaning supplies, hygiene products, toiletries, and so forth for two weeks. You should also have adequate money to pay for two weeks of living expenses without any incoming funds so that if you find yourself unable to work due to a mild emergency, you can afford to pay for your shelter and all necessary bills associated with your shelter.

The second level of preparedness is to prepare for where you will go if your home is not an option. You should know of at least one friend or family member that you can stay with in case of an emergency. Everyone in your household should see which friend or family member's house will be the designated emergency shelter. They should also know the address and the way to get there so that if everyone is not together when an emergency strikes, everyone still knows where to go so they can safely gather following the emergency.

Task 19: Shelter for Moderate to Extreme Emergency

In moderate to extreme situations, you need to have accelerated plans on how you are going to survive. You need to know where you are going to go and how that shelter is going to work for your survival. There are two options for moderate or extreme emergencies: city allocated shelters or the bush for survival in the wilderness.

Note that if you end up in a city allocated shelter or shelter that the municipality opens up during emergencies. You are not going to have full control over how you spend your time or how you contribute to your survival. In these settings, authorities will have an emergency response plan in place, and you will have to follow what they have told you to do. However, in some cases, this may be the safest course of action.

If you end up having to retreat to the bush for shelter, you are going to need to have everything on hand for survival in these situations. This includes having a BOHS location determined ahead of time, as well as all of the navigation and survival tools you will need to survive. You will need tarps, a tent if possible, ropes, stakes, ground cloth, and an ax to help create your shelter. Even if you have a pre-built shelter such as a cabin in the woods, you should still have tools on hand to create a shelter in case, for some reason, your cabin is not able to be inhabited.

In addition to all of the shelter items, make sure you have everything you need to sleep comfortably. Sleeping bags, blankets, and sleeping clothes should all be available so that you can keep yourself warm and protected during the night hours.

Task 20: Fire for Mild Emergency

Fire is responsible for both core temperature and for cooking food over in case of an emergency. If the electricity goes out, for example, a fire will allow you to keep yourself warm and continue to cook your food as usual. In a mild emergency setting, such as a down powerline or a temporary outage, you will need a way to warm yourself and your family and prepare meals for yourself at home. While a home may be more comfortable, fire can be more difficult to manage safely in urban settings.

There are three ways that you can safely bring fire indoors for warmth and cooking. They include fireplaces or wood-burning stoves, gas ranges, and candles. Fireplaces or wood-burning stoves can contain fires just as you would in the bush, which means they are incredibly useful. You will need to keep your chimney clean at all times, however, to avoid becoming poisoned by the gasses from the fireplace. If you have a gas oven or gas range, you can continue to use the elements on that range, too. Simply turn on the element and use a barbecue lighter to light the element, which will cause the gas to ignite. With gas ranges, the only part that is "off" in an outage is the electricity that powers the ignitor, and you can do that manually. Do make sure, however, that you only start it on low to avoid flame shooting out in all directions, and that you inspect gas lines for leakage before lighting any fires near your range. If there is a leakage, not only should you not light a fire but also evacuate immediately as the leak rapidly becomes fatal. For candles, you can burn as many candles as you can reasonably supervise in your home. Kerosene lamps and lanterns are also great for indoors.

Outside of your home, you can use barbecues or barbecue pits to have a fire. These are great for warming up, as well as for cooking over. Be sure to keep extra propane, charcoal blocks, or wood chips on hand so that you always have fuel for your fire. Smokers are also excellent for cooking meat if you have one, plus if you find yourself in a long term emergency, they can be used to cure meats, so they don't spoil.

Task 21: Fire for Moderate to Extreme Emergency

In moderate to extreme emergencies, you will be likely to have to procure fire outdoors. Knowing how to build and maintain a fire is crucial as it will allow you to keep yourself warm and give yourself something to cook safely. Fire crafting will require you to have a combustion tool such as a lighter or matches, access to fire starters, and fuel to supply your fire. You will also need somewhere to build it. If you are in an urban setting, fire starters can be the lint from your dryer, ripped up pieces of cardboard tubes, or cotton balls. In the wilderness, dry brush and grass, dry leaves, and pinecones are great fire starters. Fuel will virtually always be some form of dry wood, though new wood split off of a fresh tree will work in a pinch; however, you will have to be careful not to add too much, or it will drown out your fire.

There are countless fire lays you can use outdoors, though I am going to teach you the two which are most accessible and will get you furthest. These include the teepee fire lay and the Dakota pit fire lay. For either fire, you will start by cleaning off space on the ground where you can build a fire without it catching dry materials off the ground and spreading out of control. You can also shape out a fire pit using rocks, if you wish, to help contain your fire.

The teepee fire lay is created by placing fire-starting materials in the very center of your fire pit. Then, you will use kindling sized log cuts to make a small teepee over the starting materials. Do not make the teepee too dense, or oxygen will not get through and let your fire start. Next, create a giant teepee over the smaller teepee using most massive split logs or branches, which will serve as your fuel. Again, do not make them too dense, or the oxygen will not get through for your fire. Now, start the starting materials in the center. They will catch on fire, then they will catch the smaller kindling on fire, and then that will start your fuel logs going.

The Dakota pit fire lay uses two holes in the ground, and it is ideal for cooking, as well as for keeping a fire going in a windy area. You will create the Dakota fire pit by digging a small hole into the ground at least 1' deep. Then, you will dig another hole into the ground on an angle aimed at the bottom of the original hole. Do not break through with the shovel, though. Use your hand to break a hole through the bottom that is roughly the size of your fist. Now, layer starting materials in the bottom of the central hole and make a small teepee shape out of kindling over the top of the starting materials. Start the starting materials on fire, then allow them to burn up into the kindling. You should get a pretty good fire going in your pit in no time.

The secondary hole will feed oxygen into your fire, keeping it going. When you add fuel logs to your fire, make sure they are relatively small so that plenty of oxygen can still get in and around your fire.

Task 22: Food for Mild Emergency

For a mild emergency, you want to have enough food on hand for at least two weeks at any given time. This means that you should seek to stock your pantry with enough staples that you will have two weeks' worth of food stored *on top of* your average grocery shopping routine. Choose ready to eat, non-perishable food items such as canned foods or pre-packaged foods that can be cooked right away. Homemade canned goods work great, too. Ensure they are prepared properly, though, to avoid the risk of contracting botulism due to poorly preserved food. Also, choose to have pantry staples on hand that allow you to cook and bake things such as soups, bread, and other meal items. The freezer is another great place to store items, but be careful not to rely exclusively on it. If your power goes out, the contents of your freezer would be rendered useless fairly quickly. If you do have food in your freezer, be sure to have a plan for how you will use it rapidly in case something happens to your freezer. Keeping extra tools on hand for preserving foods is a good idea. You can smoke and dry excess meat and properly can fruits and vegetables out of the freezer should it become unreliable. This way, you can salvage as much as possible.

Keeping up to two weeks' worth of food on hand means that in an emergency, you have plenty of food to eat. A great example of a usage for this store would be for emergencies such as the new coronavirus. When coronavirus first hit, there was a strain on our food sources. However, many items were still available in limited quantities. Having food reserves ensures that should this happen again; you have access to what you need during that period.

Task 23: Food for Moderate to Extreme Emergency

For a moderate to an extreme emergency, you want to have food that will last you at least one month. However, many preppers argue that you should have enough staples for anywhere from 3 months to 12 months, depending on what they believe is likely going to happen. You should find the amount that feels comfortable for you and store that amount. However, it should be no less than one month's worth of food in your pantry at any given time. Again, this should be on top of your regular grocery shopping, and it should contain items that are ready to eat, as well as ingredients for greater recipes.

It is also essential that you consider your needs for food in case you have to evacuate your house. Keep some food inside your GnG bag at all times, and be prepared to add extras from your pantry if you have to evacuate in an emergency. For your GnG bag, meals that are kept in vacuum-sealed bags or pouches are ideal as they will be lightest to carry. Canned items are good as well, but stay away from most things in glass jars as these jars can break in the bag and destroy your items.

A proper trapping kit, fishing kit, and game processing tools should be in your GnG bag, too. This way, you have everything you need to harvest food when you are in the wilderness. A book about edible plants and dangerous plants in your locale would be ideal. This will also help you safely forage for vegetation so that you are not relying solely on meat in the bush. You should also have a detailed guide on how to butcher, cook, and preserve small mammals, medium mammals, birds, reptiles and amphibians, and fish in the bush. I discuss all of those details in *Survival 101: Bushcraft*.

Task 24: First Aid for Mild Emergency

First aid is essential in emergencies. Some situations become emergencies solely because someone has become ill or injured, so having proper first aid supplies on hand can help you deal with that situation. You should have a properly stocked first aid kit on hand at all times, and everyone in your house and on your A-Team should know how to use the contents of that kit.

For mild emergencies, a first aid kit should also be kept in any vehicles you own, as well as anywhere that you may frequent, such as your place of work. If you are dropping your child off somewhere such as a daycare facility on a regular basis or with a family member or friend to be watched, make sure they also have a properly stocked first aid kit for minor emergencies.

Task 25: First Aid for Moderate to Extreme Emergency

For moderate to extreme emergency situations, you need properly stocked first aid kits on hand as well as education on how to use those kits, and how to administer basic first aid support.

First, let's talk about the first aid kits you will need. You want a fully stocked first aid kit with enough supplies in it for every single person on the A-Team for your BOHS location. Then, you want smaller first aid kits that can be carried away from camp, and that should be carried away from camp *any* time someone leaves camp. This means if you leave camp to go to the cooking location, the food storage location, to get water, to go set traps, or to do anything else, you bring this first aid kit with you. The on the go first aid kit should include tools for cleaning and dressing wounds, as well as for securing broken digits or limbs. Everything else can stay back at camp.

Everyone on the A-Team should also take a first aid course to learn how to administer first aid on the scene if need be. This will help you treat yourself and treat other members of the A-Team should something go wrong. Understanding how to administer basic first aid will result in you knowing how to handle minor wounds, set broken digits or limbs, and rescue and resuscitate people. First aid courses will also educate everyone on how to safely assess dangerous situations so that they can rescue an individual without putting themselves in harm's way.

Task 26: Emergency Equipment for Work/School

Emergency equipment for work or school includes any equipment one might need to be able to complete their duty away from work or school. This is more common in mild emergencies, as more advanced emergencies would not likely allow you to continue working or completing school work as you went. For mild emergencies, however, having access to the tools you need to continue working will ensure that you can continue earning an income and that your child is able to continue advancing their education as you endure your emergency.

Task 27: Digital Copies of Important Documents

Important documents like ID, birth certificates, marriage certificates, social security numbers, insurance numbers and papers, and health ID numbers should always be kept on hand. Bank numbers, investment numbers, and other important documents should also be kept available. With that being said, the hard copies of these documents can become damaged, so you will want to keep them available in digital copies, too. To create digital copies of your important documents, be sure to upload them by scanning them to your computer. Then, e-mail them to yourself and keep them on at least two separate USB drives kept in 2 separate places. One should be in your GnG bag; the other should be kept away from the house, such as in a safety deposit box. This ensures that you always have a copy of your important documents, no matter what happens. In emergency situations, these documents are very important, so you will want to be confident that you have them, and that you know where they are.

Task 28: Travel Equipment

When preparing for a survival situation, it is important that you don't get caught up on your place of origin and your destination and forget entirely about your mode of transportation! If you will need to leave your home for survival, or if you will be away from your home and need to return, you need to have equipment on hand for traveling with. Keeping some equipment in your GnG bag, as well as in your car, is a great way to make sure that you have everything you need to travel with. If you do not have a car, keep extra cash on hand so that you can pay for transportation if need be, in more mild emergencies.

Your GnG bag should include the following travel equipment: a pair of comfortable hiking boots, a change of dry clothes, a flashlight, and extra bags to make hauling your supplies easier. If you are heading to a place with mild terrain, consider a folding wagon that can be used on back road trails, as this will take some of the weight off your back and help you get more into your camp.

Another thing to consider as far as travel equipment goes is having a travel plan. In other words, how will all members of the A-Team be traveling in an emergency situation? Which cars will be taken, who will be responsible for driving who, and how will you assign travel to each individual? Knowing where everyone will be traveling, and how, ensures that everyone is accounted for in the plan. This way, you know everyone will arrive at the BOHS safely.

Task 29: Survival Vest Equipment

Survival vests are a type of survival gear that is worn on your body and that are designed to help keep you warm, dry, and comfortable while also allowing you to bring gear along with you easily. Survival vests have multiple pockets and compartments for storing things in. The benefit of having a well-stocked vest is that you do not have to open your bag and search for things every time you are looking for something that you would commonly need on the trail. As well, if you are going to be surviving in the bush for a while, you can often carry everything you need for shorter trips in your vest and only take a few small things with you in a pack or your hands.

Your vest should always have:

- A fishing kit
- Survival blankets, an emergency blanket, and small tarps
- Map, compass, and flashlight
- Tough trash bag
- Dental floss and needles
- Small first aid kit and sanitizer
- Water purification tablets or drops
- Duct tape and cordage
- Firestarter and a lighter
- Whistle and signal mirror
- Multi-tool and knife
- Small cook pot and power bars
- Survival poncho

Task 30: Personal Equipment

Personal equipment includes everything that one person needs for survival. Since you have already addressed water, food, shelter, fire, and first aid, the next thing to address is your personal needs. Personal needs include things like clothes, toothbrushes and toothpaste, personal medications, and other personal needs you might have. If you have a child in your house, you might have a particular blanket for that child or a special stuffed animal you use to help comfort them. If you have someone who particularly likes reading, you might include a book or two in your pack if you have room, so they have something to do. While there is not a lot of downtime in the bush, having something to keep you occupied in a positive manner, such as reading or a game or pocket chess, can help keep your mind calm. This is a great way to distract yourself if you are having a hard time mentally processing the stress of being in a survival situation.

Task 31: Car Equipment

In your car, you should also have basic equipment to help you repair your car if need be. A spare tire plus everything needed to change your tire should be kept on hand, in the car, at all times. As well, flares, cones, a reflective safety jacket, extra motor oil and coolant, an emergency blanket, and a flashlight with extra batteries are all crucial to have in your car at all times. A travel-sized tool kit would also be ideal, particularly if it has screwdrivers, an adjustable wrench, pliers, and a pocket knife. Lastly, keep jumper cables on hand, which will help you jumpstart your car if need be. As well, keep your tank as close to empty at all times so that if you ever do come across an emergency, you have enough gas to get you where you need to go.

Task 32: Pre-Packaged Supplies

Pre-packaged supplies include anything you can purchase that has already been designed for you, essentially. Bushcraft and survival stores often sell kits that contain everything you need for certain aspects of living in the wilderness. For example, there may be cooking kits, personal hygiene kits, burn kits, first aid kits, fishing kits, and other such kits pre-built. These kits are excellent as they tend to come at a discounted price, are already packaged in a way that makes them easy to transport, and are often kept organized. Ensure that any pre-packaged kits have everything you need in them. Do not be afraid to add extra things to a kit if need be so that you have everything you feel you would need in a survival setting. It is better to feel confident in what you have then to rely on someone else to do the work for you. Be sure to pay attention to expiry dates on kits, as some will have expiry dates. You will need to include them in your rotation and inspection so that you can replace anything that expires.

Task 33: GnG Bag for Mild Emergency

Your GnG bag for mild emergencies should be full of everything you would need in an emergency at home or close to home. The bag should contain everything you would need in a mild emergency. Your A-Team contact sheet, water, prevention checklists, food, and a first aid kit should all be kept in the mild GnG bag.

Keeping everything in a GnG bag, even if it will only be used at home, means that you can quickly grab it and bring it to the scene of an emergency and promptly use anything you need. You can also keep this bag near your moderate to extreme GnG bag as you will want to take it with you in a moderate or extreme situation, too.

Task 34: GnG Bag for Moderate to Extreme Emergency

Your moderate to extreme emergency GnG bag should contain absolutely everything you would need to survive any emergency. This includes all of your Bushcraft gear, plus everything you would need for food, water, shelter, fire, and first aid in a moderate to extreme emergency situation. These should be kept next to your GnG bag for mild situations so that you can grab all of your GnG bags and get out as soon as you can. Make sure all of your GnG bags are easily accessible, well-stocked, and organized in a way that makes it easy for you to access anything you may need in any situation you may happen upon.

CHAPTER 6

How To Leave An Urban Environment

Leaving an urban environment may sound easy in theory, but the reality is that if you are going to survive after you leave, you are going to have to know what you are doing. Urban living is much different from rural living, and even more different from living in the wilderness. Be ready to not only access your survival environment but to navigate it as well.

There are five things you must do if you are going to safely leave an urban environment and successfully survive in a rural or wilderness environment. These include: preparing your supplies, plotting your destination, educating yourself on your destination, learning skills ahead of time, and securing the first 5 of survival.

Preparing Your Supplies

Before you ever leave your urban environment, you will first need to prepare your supplies. Have your GnG bags packed, survival vest available, and everything ready to go at all times. In an urban environment, you have far greater access to the tools, supplies, and resources that you will need to survive in the bush, so you will want to collect these before leaving.

Moderate to extreme emergencies that require you to leave urban environments often make it so that you are unable to access supplies, as well. For example, a hurricane would shut down all of the grocery stores and gas stations in your area as everyone runs to protect themselves. Do not wait until an emergency strikes to prepare these supplies. Otherwise, you will find yourself struggling to get anything at all. Supplies may become inaccessible, they will sell out quickly, and accessing them even if they are available could become dangerous. Further, having to stop to get supplies first wastes your precious time that could instead be spent getting away to your BOHS location. Having them on hand is the only sure way to ensure that you have what you need and that you can escape to safety as quickly as possible.

Again, always check your supplies every 6-12 months and never leave supplies wiped out. If you use anything out of your first aid kit, for example, make sure you promptly replace it. Or, if you find yourself using things regularly, such as bandages, keep a different box for the house and a separate pack for the GnG bag. That way, you always have some on hand in your emergency bag. This is the only way to ensure that when you find yourself in an emergency, you have everything you need available for you right away.

Plotting Your Destination

You should never leave an urban environment without first knowing where you are going. Having a BOHS identified in advance ensures that you know exactly where to head in case of a moderate to extreme emergency situation. Driving aimlessly out of the city with no clear destination is a sure way to find yourself in potentially even more of a dangerous situation than you were already in.

Even during every day settings, the safest driving technique is to go directly from route A to route B. Naturally, the less time spent on the road, the less you are endangered by your moving vehicle or other moving vehicles. Now let's consider an emergency situation. In an emergency situation, no matter how level-headed you tend to be, you are going to be under stress. Further, there is no way to know whether or not the road to safety is available, or if any of your backup routes are accessible, either. Ultimately, you are hopeful that you are heading to safety, but you may still run into troubles along the way. If you do not know where you are going, you increase the amount of time you spend on a potentially dangerous road that you are unfamiliar with. This can also increase your stress levels, making driving even more dangerous.

You should always identify your BOHS location in advance and have a secondary BOHS location available in case the first one does not work out. This way, you can feel confident that you know where you are going and how to get there. There is no increased risk of you being on the road too long, or heading to a location you are not familiar with.

Educating Yourself on Your Destination

Beyond knowing what your specific destination is, you also need to educate yourself on your specific destination. Educate yourself on everything that would be relevant to you surviving in this location, *and* get out there and see it for yourself. Surviving on assumptions is never a good idea; you want certainty and confidence in your survival situation.

While educating yourself on your BOHS destination, start by educating yourself on exactly how to get there. Look for a direct route, as well as alternate routes. Then, educate yourself on what methods will be required for you to get to that location. Will you be able to drive straight in? Or are you going to have to park your car lower down and walk into the proper camping area?

You will need to educate yourself about the environment itself, too. Are you going to a space that is occupied by the desert? Wetlands? Tundra? Consider the climate, the geography, and what the terrain itself is like. How easy is it to move around in this terrain? What types of threats, dangers, or other things do you need to consider when walking in this area? Will you need to cut out paths? And if so, how will you do it? Consider everything you will need to know for getting there, setting up, and navigating the terrain as you survive in this location.

Lastly, educate yourself on the vegetation, insects, and animals in that area. What plants are you likely to come across? Take note of which plants are useful, which are edible, and which plants are dangerous. Keep a book handy, so you can educate yourself in the field, rather than trying to rely on memory when you are already stressed. Consider the insects, as well. Some insects will be harmless, but some may be dangerous. How can you protect yourself against pests to avoid being contaminated with a disease or affected by a venomous bite? Then, think about wildlife. What types of critters are you likely to come across? Which can be eaten, which can be ignored, and which are considered threats or dangers to your wellbeing?

After you have educated yourself on everything, prepare yourself to deal with it all, too. Customize your GnG bags and survival gear to suit the terrain, the vegetation, the animals, and the likely tasks you will have to engage in so that you can survive in that area. Get out in the field and actually visit that area, too, to ensure your assumptions are correct and your preparations are on par for the environment. The more prepared you are, the better your chances of survival will be.

Learning Skills In Advance

In addition to preparing your supplies in advance, you should also focus on learning skills in advance, too. At least, learn as many as you reasonably can. Educate yourself on what skills will be necessary to your survival and begin to discover how you can master those skills, even while living in an urban environment. Some you may be able to practice at home or in your urban setting, while others you may benefit from going camping in a region similar to your BOHS location, or in your BOHS location specifically. Do whatever you can to learn as much as possible beforehand so that when you arrive in the field in a survival emergency, you are safe and ready to face that emergency situation in every way possible.

Some of the skills you might consider learning in advance are in the five main areas of your survival, including water, food, shelter, fire, and first aid. Below, you will find some skills you should start focusing on developing right away.

- Water: how to find water, how to treat water, how to test the water, how to store water.
- Food: how to cook different basic recipes, how to set up a trap, how to fish, how to find bait, how to track animals, how to preserve animals, how to forage, how to identify edible plants from toxic plants, how to store food safely in a campsite.
- Shelter: how to build a tent, how to make a tent out of a tarp, how to make a shelter out of all natural items (branches, brush, leaves, grasses, etc.), how to insulate a shelter, how to check the environment for a safe location to build a shelter.
- Fire: how to identify different pieces of wood, how to locate wood, how to cut wood, how to split wood, how to make a basic fire lay, how to make a fire starter, how to start a fire, how to fuel a fire, how to safely cook over a fire.
- First aid: how to pack a first aid kit, how to use the different elements of a first aid kit, how to dress a wound, how to treat a burn, how to treat gastrointestinal issues, local plants with medicinal values, how to make a poultice, how to set a bone, how to transport someone who is unable to move, how to resuscitate someone.

Securing the First 5 of Survival

The first five of survival include water, food, shelter, fire, and first aid or safety. These are used to help secure your core temperature and provide you with everything you need in order to survive. If you set yourself up well, they are also set up in a way that amplifies your comfort and convenience, which makes survival a lot easier. In an urban setting, you are likely already educated on how to secure these five elements of your wellbeing. In an off-grid survival situation, these five elements change a bit, though.

Water is not fetched from a tap or a store, but instead from a water source. You need to be prepared to locate a water source, carry water back to camp, treat the water, and drink it. Store water in stainless steel containers that have been sterilized in boiling water and cooled completely to avoid burning yourself.

Food is not fetched from a store, either. You are going to need to be able to track food sources and trap or fish for those sources so that you can bring meat back to camp. Protein and fat are essential staples of a survivalists diet as it provides you with the best energy to keep you going. Most of your calories are burnt when resting, so when you are in a situation where you need to take action, you will *definitely* need to prepare yourself by bulking up on as much protein and fat as possible. You also need to learn how to safely forage for food, clean food, and consume food from plant life in the local area.

Shelter is not put in place, nor can you hire a building crew to build your shelter. You are going to need to know how to fly a tarp, how to set up a tent, how to build a shelter, and where to build a shelter. You are also going to need to know how to make sure that the shelter is waterproof and warm so that you do not risk yourself by remaining too wet or by cooling down too much on cooler days or nights.

Fire is not something that can easily be created through candles, fireplaces, gas ranges, or barbecues when you are surviving in the woods. You need to know how to make a fire lay, start a fire, and maintain a fire. You are also going to need to know how to safely cook on the fire so that you do not burn yourself, but you can consume the food you have harvested safely.

Lastly, backwoods first aid is different from urban first aid because you do not have immediate access to trained medical staff or sterilized medical equipment that can be used in any emergency or first aid situation. Even if you are in a situation where you can call the authorities for assistance, there is no guarantee that they will get there in time. You will need to know how to treat all minor injuries and illnesses and how to address all major injuries and illnesses until you can get the help of a medical professional. If you have escaped to live off-grid because authorities are a danger to you and your family, you might have to learn to do even more first aid so you can adequately deal with emergencies in the bush, without help.

Practice Evacuations

Everything always works perfectly in theories. In practical application is where you begin to run into trouble with any plans you may have prepared for yourself and your family. An essential step to preparing yourself to leave an urban environment is practicing your evacuation ahead of time when no pressing emergency is present. Practice evacuations ensure that you have a concise and realistic understanding of what is required during a real evacuation and allows you to create an evacuation protocol that actually works.

Ensure that your household and any other households involved in your A-Team practice evacuations every so often to ensure you are all prepared for a real evacuation, should one be required. It may feel silly to practice escaping when no threat is looming, but understand that this critical step can help you recognize weaknesses in your plan and offset them with plan adjustments ahead of time. This way, during a real threat, your evacuation plan works, and everyone safely arrives at your ERP, or IRP, depending on the type of evacuation being practiced.

An effective way to practice an evacuation would be to first compose a theory of how your evacuation should look. Then, create a theoretical emergency and form a "sudden call" to the A-Team of this emergency. Immediately, everyone should enact the evacuation protocol and begin fulfilling their role in that protocol. The practice drill is over when everyone meets at the ERP or the IRP, depending on the drill being practiced. Immediately after, everyone should reflect on how the practice drill went, and what could have improved the quality of the evacuation. Attempt to imagine additional challenges that may have been imposed due to emergencies, as well, to get a clearer understanding of how safety during the evacuation can be secured. Practice your adjusted drill until you have reached the point where you have an evacuation protocol that works.

Practice your final evacuation protocol at least once per year once it has been finalized. This ensures that as things change, such as someone moves, someone is no longer physically capable, or new people join the A-Team; these changes are accommodated for in your evacuation protocol. Adequate, up-to-date preparedness will always ensure the smoothest possible escape from a dangerous emergency at any given time, so take this step seriously and practice it frequently.

CHAPTER 7
Long Term Off-Grid Survival

If you find yourself needing to survive off-grid for a long time, you are going to need to acquire additional skills that will allow you to secure your survival for extended periods. Knowing what no respite is coming and that you have to fend for yourself for extended periods can be frightening. Still, it is entirely possible and can be done successfully. As long as you are prepared to learn the necessary skills and implement the required steps, a human can survive through just about anything.

Foraging and Scavenging In Natural Environments

Procuring food in natural environments is not always easy, but it is necessary. You cannot live solely off of game meat for survival, especially over long periods of time, as you expose yourself to many different types of illnesses. Humans require a number of vitamins that come from plant matter to be able to maintain a healthy immune system, which will, in turn, fend off any illness and help with faster healing.

Foraging and scavenging in natural environments depend on what environment you are living in. If you are living long term, you are going to want to have enough food available to help you through periods where food may be more challenging to get. For example, in most areas, winters are particularly challenging because they are cooler, and many animals stop reproducing, go into hibernation, and generally lay low for the season. As well, hunting in winter seasons is more challenging because of the snow and the cold. Having a regular system for foraging, scavenging, and hunting will ensure that you have enough food to last you.

Raised Bed Gardening

One way you can secure food for yourself, and the A-Team is to engage in raised bed gardening. Raised bed gardening can be done at home or off-grid and can be incredibly helpful in keeping enough food available for you and your family. When it comes to raised bed gardening, you need to think about growing hardy crops that are going to get you the furthest and that are able to handle harsher growing conditions. This way, if you have a rough growing season, you are still likely to get some food out of it. You should also grow foods that preserve well as it is unlikely that you will be able to consume all that food at once. Further, it would be unwise of you to grow plenty of food only to have none of it last through until the end of winter.

Another thing you are going to have to consider with raised bed gardening is the element of competition. Pests such as insects, rodents, birds, small mammals, and even some medium and large mammals can come through and destroy any crop in a matter of hours. You need to have a method in place for protecting your crop, while also having a method in place for harvesting fresh produce before anyone else gets to it. I talk more about the specifics of raised bed gardening in *Survival 101: Raised Bed Gardening*.

Long Term Food Preservation

Long term food preservation will ensure that you always have an abundance of food, even during seasons where gathering food may be more challenging. There are many different methods of long term food preservation, all of which can be useful in preserving your harvest through slow seasons. Canning is perhaps the most popular method of preservation when it comes to things like fruits and vegetables. However, your ability to can will depend on whether or not you were able to bring any canning supplies with you. If you can, have a proper canning guide on hand, too. A proper book will educate you on how to safely can all of your supplies to avoid accidental illness or death due to botulism.

Drying out and dehydrating fruit and vegetables is another great way to preserve your harvest. This can be done with minimal equipment, and the food can be consumed dry or rehydrated at a later point with filtered water when you are cooking.

Drying, salting, and smoking meat are all the best methods for preserving meat when you are in the wilderness. These methods will ensure that your meat is safe so that you can consume it at a later date. I discuss more food preservation in *Survival 101: Food Storage*.

Preparing for Climate Changes

If you are going to be surviving in the wilderness for an extended period, you are going to need to know how to prepare for climate change. The general way the seasons of survival in the wilderness go include: spring – start the harvest, summer, – grow the harvest, fall – preserve the harvest, and winter, – consume the harvest. You will need to prepare in other ways, too. For summer, you will want to prepare for animals awakening, bugs becoming more active, and more bacteria and viruses waking up. In the winter, you want to prepare for how much more challenging it will be for you to access food and water sources by having plenty on hand for you to consume.

You will also want to prepare your shelter for climate change. In the summer, you will want to do what you can to keep your shelter cooler so that you do not overheat in it, while during winter months, you are going to want to insulate your shelter so that you stay warmer.

Building Long Term Shelter

Long term shelter is going to be necessary if you are going to be surviving somewhere for a lengthy period. While tarp shelters and tents are great for short term survival, they will not suffice if you need to be anywhere for a longer period. Over longer periods, these shelters become a risk because they are able to tear, they are not as easy to keep warm, and they do not do a particularly good job at keeping predators and pests out. Building long term shelter will ensure that you have everything you need to keep yourself safe and healthy for long periods.

Long term shelter should consider longevity, security, and all of your fundamental needs. It should be built in a way that is lasting, that keeps animals out to the best of your ability, and that makes doing things like storing your goods, cooking, and doing other such things much easier. You may want to build a long term sleeping cabin, as well as a food cabin and a storage cabin a ways away from your sleeping cabin. This way, you can safely protect all of your belongings while still following proper practice to protect yourself, too.

Navigating Disasters

Navigating disasters in the wilderness may seem challenging. Things like financial collapses will not affect your living in the wilderness; however, they may drive you there. Preparing for a financial collapse is best done by storing as much as you possibly can, and learning how to grow and harvest more so that you can rely on yourself for subsistence. This way, if the financial collapse occurs and money becomes worthless, you can still protect your survival. Another situation that may completely block you from being able to access what you need would be offense warfare attacks. Some places are prone to attacks by opposing armies or by civil armies in the case of civil warfare. In these circumstances, if you go off-grid, you want to stay in hiding to avoid anyone infiltrating you and destroying your survival situation.

Pandemics are tough to deal with. Early on, you may have access to all of your normal supply chains, but as pandemics, rage on it can become increasingly more dangerous to live in an urban environment and interact with other people. Moving your A-Team away to an off-grid situation and avoiding or eliminating contact with the outside world is a great way to prevent yourself and the A-Team from contracting the pandemic virus. Many believe that an illness may one day come through and wipe out civilization, which is why they prepare, and these individuals live as off-grid as possible to avoid coming into contact with any such pandemics, and ultimately dying.

Natural disasters can lead to short and long term survival situations. When they involve financial collapse, for example, they end up becoming long term survival situations. Regardless of how your home may come back together, the recession it leaves your region in can be devastating. In a natural disaster, you should be aware of how the disaster affects your home, your travel route, and your BOHS location. Act accordingly. If it is unsafe for you to stay home or go to the BOHS location, rely on an alternate plan to protect yourself and the A-Team.

The best way to navigate disasters is to plan for them and to create a clear plan for how you will deal with any such disaster. You should also have back up plans for what you are going to do if your ideal plans do not turn out. As well, you should educate yourself on what it is like to attempt to survive such a disaster so that you are prepared for what may be expected of you in order for survival to even be possible. Always plan and prepare for the worst in survival situations, so you have everything you need to survive anything that happens to you. That way, you always have the best chance of survival.

CHAPTER 8

Emergency And First Aid

Dealing with emergencies and first aid situations in the bush can be scary. In some cases, it may be possible for you to deal with them yourself. With others, you may need to contact support to assist you with the situation you have found yourself in. There are some general guidelines you should follow to help you make your judgment call. Still, at the end of the day, you are going to need to decide what is right for the situation you are in and go from there.

When to Contact the Police

In mild emergencies, contacting the police or your local emergency line is a great way to get access to help. In moderate to extreme emergencies, calling the police should be something you do only if you need to. The reason behind this is that you do not want to contact the police and overburden their system with calls from a local emergency. Alternatively, you do not wish to contact the police and rely on them if they are going to be a danger to you or your family.

More recently, the threat of places turning into a police state has become more significant than ever. That threat means that not everyone can rely on the local police force. When a police state is enacted, none of us may be able to genuinely rely on the police force because it operates on a different agenda. Trusting in them could lead to imprisonment or even death in some cases. If you are in a situation where you have escaped from a police state or where you are likely to be harmed by the police, you should refrain from calling the cops and instead have a support group of people you can call on for assistance in emergencies. This counts whether you are still in urban civilization, or if you have evacuated to the bush to survive off-grid due to an emergency you may be facing.

When to Contact FEMA

FEMA, or the Federal Emergency Management Agency, is located in the Department of Homeland Security. They are responsible for coordinating the federal government's response to natural and man-made disasters. In some situations, FEMA can be incredibly helpful with a disaster you may be facing. FEMA can also help deal with acts of terror, allowing them to provide a great deal of support to anyone who may be facing a disaster.

You should only contact FEMA if you have faced an emergency, and if you feel confident, they can help. If, however, you are someone who is likely to be questioned or imprisoned by the government, calling FEMA may not be a good idea. At times, particularly when a police state is enacted, relying on any government infrastructure may be dangerous. If you have any reason to believe you would be put at risk, avoid relying on FEMA, and instead navigate the disaster using your own survival skills and supplies.

Utilizing Government Infrastructure

Relying on government infrastructure is something that you need to consider, particularly when there is a great deal of mistrust in the government deeply. At this time, as we face challenges with the coronavirus pandemic, many people do not trust the government and fear what may happen if they do. This can make trusting government infrastructure fearsome, especially if you believe they are intentionally engaging in wrongdoings.

Ultimately, if you are in an emergency where you believe the government themselves are unreliable and are a threat, you need to use your best judgment and avoid infrastructure at all costs. Do everything you can to survive on your own, and only call for support or rely on government infrastructure if there is absolutely no other chance. Even then, do so in a way that minimizes the risk of you and everyone you are surviving with. For example, if you are in a situation where you are surviving off-grid to avoid a police state, but someone in your camp is extremely hurt, you should bring that person down into civility and contact support for them. Then, to the best of your ability, get away from that location, and let them get help. This way, anyone who may need it can access support, but the rest of the A-Team remains safe and away from the risk of being found or harmed.

If there is no police state enacted, and there is no overarching reason to believe the government is a direct threat to you, use your best judgment. Always do what you can to only use government infrastructure when it is required, and do your best to rely on yourself and the A-Team as much as possible. This keeps you out of the government's crosshairs and in a safer position to protect yourself and other members of the A-Team.

First Aid Methods You Should Know

One of the best ways you can protect the A-Team and minimize reliance on government infrastructure is to learn how to treat minor things yourself at home or at the BOHS location. These basic first aid methods ensure that you are able to treat minor conditions in people so that they do not have to rely on government infrastructure. If treated effectively, their condition should improve, and you should be able to keep them out of the system. The three things you should know how to do on the field include dressing a wound, treating gastrointestinal illness, and dealing with broken bones.

Dressing a Wound

To dress a wound, start by cleansing the wound using an antiseptic cleaner, which will sterilize the wound from any bacteria that may have broken the skin barrier. If the injury is deep enough, you will need to sew it together using a sterile needle and medical thread. Next, you should use medical glue, medical tape, or pine resin in a pinch, to "glue" the wound together, especially if it is an unusually large wound. Even smaller wounds can use these to create a protective barrier between the injury and the external world, while the wound itself is healing. Once done, you should place clean gauze over the wound and secure it in place. Then, prevent the wound from being rubbed or aggravated by any external sources. Replace the dressing every 4-6 hours to avoid bacteria getting into the wound and causing illness through the wound itself.

Treating a Gastrointestinal Illness

A gastrointestinal illness may be bothersome in an urban environment, but in a survival environment, they can be fatal. Treating them promptly avoids someone becoming dehydrated or malnourished and ensures that they have a better chance of survival. Start by making sure that the affected person has access to clean water and high-quality protein. Sipping water and slowly snacking on dried meat is a great way to keep them hydrated and nourished. Next, you should use medicine to help treat the gastrointestinal illness. If you have any medicine on hand, use that. Otherwise, use the inner bark from a sassafras tree or a white oak tree to make a tea and consume that to treat any gastrointestinal illnesses. If sassafras or white oak do not grow in your area, educate yourself on alternative remedies that you can locate in your region's natural flora. Use this knowledge to improvised based on your current location.

Dealing With a Broken Bone

Broken bones can be incredibly dangerous in a wilderness survival location. The scent of blood from the wound can attract wildlife, and the bone itself can make saving yourself far more challenging. If a bone is completely broken or protruding, the only thing you can do is wrap the injury with a soft padded blanket and get that person to trained medical staff as soon as possible.

If a bone is fractured but not completely broken and has not broken surface, you may be able to deal with it at camp. For digits, for example, you can wrap them against a small branch so that the branch holds them straight and steady while they are healing. For legs, a larger branch can be secured to the limb to encourage the limb to heal. The limb should also be carefully wrapped to keep it protected. There should be plenty of protection between the limb and the branch to avoid wounds from rubbing. If it is an arm that is broken, a splint may be the best option for healing the broken arm. You could also attach a branch to the arm to keep it straight and sturdy, again keeping plenty of padding between the arm and the branch to avoid wounds from rubbing.

CONCLUSION

Surviving a dangerous situation seems like a nightmare. For most people, they will never actually have to live through it. For many, however, emergencies strike and lead to them having to protect themselves and fend for themselves. This may only be for the foreseeable future, or for the long haul, depending on the type of disaster they have found themselves in.

The thing about emergencies is that we never expect them, and if we do, we never expect them to be *that* bad. When they do strike, however, they can rapidly catch us off guard and leave us in a do-or-die situation. The only way to protect yourself against emergencies entails assuming that you will inevitably face one at some point in your life and prepare accordingly. You can do this by preparing yourself for mild, moderate, and extreme emergencies. If anything does happen, you are fully equipped.

As you continue to prepare for emergencies, I encourage you to keep *Survival 101: Beginner's Guide 2021* available for you to access at all times. Use this book to help you review your 34 tasks and run your rotation and inspection checklist. As well, use it to help guide you through the tasks that you may need to enact if and when you find yourself in an emergency setting. It is important that you assume that any stress you face during an emergency will disrupt your memory. Keeping clear guides on what to do ensures that should this happen, you have everything you need to stay focused and survive. Having this book printed and available in your GnG bag helps. I also encourage you to keep printed copies of *Survival 101: Bushcraft, Survival 101: Food Storage,* and *Survival 101: Raised Bed Gardening for Beginners* on hand. All four of these books will serve you massively if you ever find yourself in a survival situation.

Don't stop here, either. Continue educating yourself on what it takes to survive. Study your local environment, learn new skills, and prepare yourself in a hands-on way so that if and when you find yourself in this situation, you are ready. When it comes to your survival, you are ultimately responsible. While urban environments may be comfortable, avoid becoming complacent. Not educating yourself on survival techniques is foolish and dangerous, and can ultimately lead to illness, injuries, or fatalities during an emergency.

Before you go, I want to ask one favor. If you could please review *Survival 101: Beginner's Guide 2021*, I would greatly appreciate it. Your honest review will help others discover this great title, while also helping me create more great titles for you.

Thank you, and best of luck! Stay safe out there.

www.ingramcontent.com/pod-product-compliance
Lightning Source LLC
Chambersburg PA
CBHW081743100526
44592CB00015B/2279